MULTIDISCIPLINARY COMPETENCY ASSESSMENT:

ENSURING STAFF PERFORMANCE

BY

Janice M. Crabill, MSN, RN
Dorothy H. Mundy, MN, RN
Angel Piombino, MS, RNC, CNA
Roberta A. Raymond, MSN, RN
Carol Ann Rooks, PhD, RN

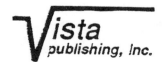

Vista publishing, inc.

Copyright © 1995 by Mercy Medical Center

All rights reserved. No part of this book may be reproduced or transmitted in any form or by any means, graphic, electronic, including photocopying, recording, or any information storage or retrieval system, for sale, without written permission from Mercy Medical Center, Center for Research, Education and Development, except as indicated in the text and with reference to the duplication of competency worksheets and forms described by the authors.

Edited by Joseph Jaeger

Cover Design by Thomas Taylor of Thomcatt Graphics

Vista Publishing, Inc.
473 Broadway
Long Branch, NJ 07740
(908) 229-6500

This publication is written for the information and education of the general public who have an interest in Competency Assessment Planning processes. The authors are solely responsible for the content of the written work and have made every effort to be accurate and up to date with all information presented. It is recommended that the reader consult other texts and reference regulations as they specifically relate to their individual institutions.

Printed and bound in the United States of America

First Edition

ISBN: 1-880254-30-1

Library of Congress Catalog Card Number: 95-60800

U.S.A. Price $85.00
Canada Price $110.50

ACKNOWLEDGMENT

As with any endeavor of this type, many people have contributed to the completion of this book.

Our colleagues, the clinical staff of Mercy Medical Center, have shared their clinical knowledge and expertise with us. They willingly participated in the development of competencies for their respective departments. The competencies that are contained in this book represent the best clinical expertise in the field.

A very special thank you to Kelly Dougherty for her secretarial support to us throughout this process.

Jan Crabill
Dot Mundy
Angel Piombino
Roberta Raymond
Carol Ann Rooks

Baltimore, Maryland
December, 1994

MEET THE AUTHORS

Janice M. Crabill, MSN, RN has more than 10 years experience in nursing education and staff development. As a Professional Development Coordinator in the Center for Research, Education, and Development at Mercy Medical Center in Baltimore, Maryland, Jan has been responsible for developing and implementing the Mother/Baby cross-training program, a mandatory educational effort on nursing assessment, and the nursing competency assessment program. She currently coordinates the Occupational Safety and Health Act (OSHA) education program and hospital orientation for the entire Medical Center. Jan is a consultant within the Medical Center, active in curriculum design and implementation, adult teaching strategies, and competency-based education.

Jan holds a Bachelor of Science in Nursing from Boston University, a Bachelor of Arts in Sociology from Eastern Nazarene College, and a Master of Science in Nursing from the Catholic University of America in Curriculum and Instruction of Maternal-Infant Nursing. Jan is currently a Doctoral Candidate in the Department of Human Development at the University of Maryland.

Dorothy H. Mundy, MN, RN is a Professional Development Coordinator in the Center for Research, Education, and Development at Mercy Medical Center in Baltimore, Maryland. Her clinical background is in high-risk obstetrical nursing and newborn intensive care. Dot has over 20 years of experience in Baccalaureate nursing education and staff development. Most recently she has been involved in the education and cross-training of the multi-skilled worker in the development of a Patient Focused Care Model of patient care delivery.

Ms. Mundy holds a Master of Nursing with a Clinical Specialty focus from the University of Florida and has completed 30 doctoral credits in Curriculum and Instruction at the University of Maryland.

Angel Piombino, MS, RNC, CNA is currently the Manager for the Center for Research, Education, and Development at Mercy Medical Center in Baltimore, Maryland. Angel has over 15 years experience in a variety of healthcare administrative and staff development settings. She holds a Master of Science in Healthcare Administration from Towson State University and certification from the American Nurses Association in both Nursing Administration and Staff Development. Angel has volunteered extensively with the American Cancer Society in the area of professional education.

Roberta A. Raymond, MSN, RN is a Professional Development Coordinator in the Center for Research, Education, and Development at Mercy Medical Center in Baltimore, Maryland. She has over 10 years of experience in nursing education and staff development. Roberta's clinical background is in the area of psychiatric/mental health nursing. She is active in the Continuous Quality Improvement Initiative at the Medical Center. Roberta coordinates the Patient Focused Care program which was recently developed at the Medical Center.

Roberta holds a Master of Science in Nursing and a Master of Arts in Education form West Virginia University and is currently a Doctoral Candidate at the University of Maryland at Baltimore. She is a member of Sigma Theta Tau, Inc., Alpha Rho Chapter.

Carol Ann Rooks, PhD, RN is a Professional Development Coordinator with 15 years of experience in trauma and critical care nursing. Carol Ann has taught undergraduate and graduate nurses at both the University of North Carolina at Chapel Hill and the University of Maryland. She holds a Master of Science in Nursing in Trauma and Critical Care and a Doctorate in Nursing and Health Care Ethics.

Special Note: The authors of *The Multidisciplinary Competency Assessment: Ensuring Staff Performance* are available for consultative services. They may be reached by telephone at (410) 332-9071 or, by mail by writing to: Mercy Medical Center
Center for Research, Education and Development
301 Saint Paul Place
Baltimore, Maryland 21202-2165

FORWARD

The Mission Statement of Mercy Medical Center promises patients and their families "excellent clinical services within a community of compassionate care . . . ." Furthermore, Mercy's philosophy contains *excellence* and *empowerment* as two of the organization's core values. *Excellence* brings us to the highest standards of clinical care; *empowerment* frees us to act, on our own behalf and on the behalf of others, to achieve excellence. These two values are fundamental to both the purpose and the content of ***Multidisciplinary Competency Assessment: Ensuring Staff Performance.***

The Nursing Competency Assessment Program originated at Mercy in response to the Joint Commission on Accreditation of Healthcare Organizations and other regulatory standards. However, as Mercy, along with all health care organizations, has been experiencing growing competitive pressure to excel financially as well as clinically, the drive for consistently high performance from all clinical staff has become more compelling. Today, the Multidisciplinary Competency Assessment Program is an integral part of Mercy's strategy to ensure excellence in clinical care and success in this competitive health care business environment.

The Professional Development staff of the Center for Research, Education and Development at Mercy Medical Center present this publication as a template for competency assessment. The authors discuss relevant regulatory standards, guide the reader through development of a competency program, outline department-specific competency plans and provide actual competency worksheets. It is our hope that, like Mercy, other health care organizations will realize clinical and competitive benefits through multidisciplinary competency assessment.

Sr. Helen Amos
Chief Executive Office
Mercy Medical Center

Amy E. Freeman
Senior Vice President
Mercy Medical Center

PREFACE

We first began to develop a Competency Assessment Program during the summer of 1993. Over 250 hours were utilized to develop the initial 90 competencies used by the Department of Nursing. Since 1993 our program has expanded to include most of the departments in the Patient Care Services division of Mercy Medical Center in Baltimore, Maryland. This division includes those departments with direct patient intervention, including Respiratory Therapy, Nutrition, and Physical Therapy, among others. We plan to implement the program in all departments in the hospital by Fall, 1995. The competencies included in this book are not intended to be inclusive of every skill or knowledge base which may need to assessed, but will provide a broad cross-section of competencies by clinical area.

Several times since the program began, remarks have been made concerning how helpful it would be if other staff development specialists were able to implement the program without having to "reinvent the wheel." We hope that this book will be used by others in the development of their competency assessment programs. Although the material is copyrighted, the authors grant permission to institutions who buy the book to utilize the worksheets or forms in their entirety for the development of a similar program.

The Authors

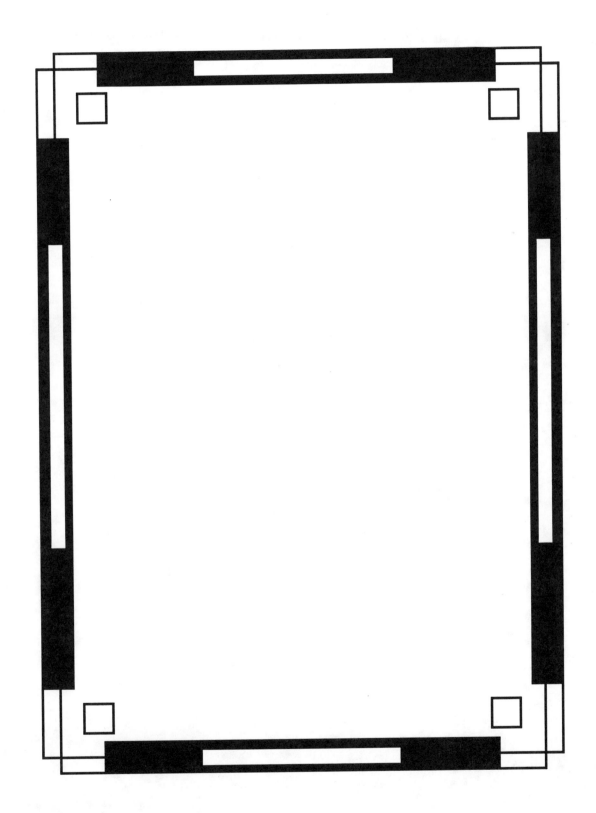

CONTENTS

CHAPTER 1

DEFINITIONS OF COMPETENCE

Chapter 1

DEFINITIONS OF COMPETENCE

In addition to providing multidisciplinary, cost-conscious approaches to patient care, all departments within the health care facility are accountable for providing evidence that individual staff members have adequate knowledge and skills to **perform** their designated job responsibilities. This process of providing evidence of ability to perform job responsibilities has been identified as performance-based evaluation, criterion-referencing, and competency assessment (Kemp, 1985). Due to the emergence of competency assessment as the term of choice utilized by the Joint Commission on Accreditation of Healthcare Organizations (JCAHO) and by seminar leaders, Mercy Medical Center has chosen to utilize the latter term to describe its ongoing program of ensuring staff performance.

The term **clinically competent** describes the individual who is fully capable of independently and correctly performing the roles and responsibilities associated with a specific position in a specific setting. Common synonyms for this term include proficiency and mastery. Although historically competence has been defined and tested in terms of knowledge, Morgan and Irby (1978) explained that the competent individual must possess both knowledge and clinical skills. The focus of **competency assessment** is on "the ability to perform a task or behavior correctly rather than on the ability to demonstrate knowledge" (Stewart & Vitello-Cicciu, 1989, p. 34). It compares behavioral performance of ability by an individual to previously established performance standards.

Competence incorporates both measurable and intangible abilities. The abilities and behaviors which can be measured through direct performance are collectively called **competencies** or singly - a **competency** (Alspach, 1993; Robinson & Barberis-Ryan, 1995). Alspach (1993) defined a competency as "an intellectual, attitudinal, or motor capability." Del Bueno, Weeks, and Brown-Stewart (1987) warned against simply replacing the term skill or ability with the term competency, stating that each competency consists of interpersonal and critical thinking components as well as technical skills. We believe that the intangible components of competence such as risk-taking, conceptualization, and use of intuition may not be observed in any one specific testing situation but become evident over time. Consistent practice of measurable competent behaviors and use of these intangible components contribute to the identification of an individual as proficient.

The concept of competence has been widely addressed in the nursing literature since the late 1970s when programs on competency-based orientations (CBO) for the service arena and competency-based education (CBE) for the academic arena were presented (Del Bueno, 1984). The competency efforts in the early 1980s, derived from these seminars (Del Bueno, 1984; O'Grady & O'Brien, 1992), attempted to address the problem of orientation plans which made no distinction between experienced nurses who needed brief orientations and novices who required extended orientations. By the mid-1980s, most nursing orientations were built upon the concept of competency, using preceptorships and performance criteria to evaluate new staff members, but the criteria did not consistently validate actual performance (DiMauro & Mack, 1989; Lawinger, 1991). Most programs relied on competencies identified by experts in the field rather than by observation and description of actual clinical activities (Benner, 1982). Many competency-based programs to date continue to address issues related to orientation and to roles and responsibilities of new staff members (DiMauro & Mack, 1989; Lawinger, 1991; Peterson, 1991; Schmaus, 1987; Selfridge, 1984).

Beginning in the late 1980s, regulatory agencies such as the Joint Commission on the Accreditation of Healthcare Organizations (JCAHO) and laws such as the Clinical Laboratory Improvement Act of 1988 (CLIA '88) have given new emphasis to competency-based evaluation of staff members. Competency assessment is mandated by the 1995 JCAHO Human Resources standard HR.3, which requires that "the competence of all staff members is assessed, maintained, demonstrated, and improved on an **ongoing basis**" (p. 52). This new feature of the standard requires that competency be assessed at periodic intervals rather than just at the beginning of a career or entry into a new organization. The standard allows each individual institution to define intervals to be used for the assessment of competence.

Aside from compliance with the standards of regulatory agencies, implementation of an ongoing competency assessment program provides additional benefits to the health care facility. Trautman and Watson (1995) identified four positive outcomes of an ongoing competency assessment program for Emergency Department nurses, including:

* facilitation of individual professional development,
* enhancement of accountability and autonomy for nurses,
* promotion of cost-effective quality patient care, and
* improved patient outcomes.

Goltz, Johnsen, and Johnson (1984) identified several positive outcomes of the ongoing competency assessment program for staff nurses in a psychiatric hospital. Their program assured that "only competent and credentialed professionals would be performing certain aspects of patient care" (p.44). This assurance led to a greater team cohesiveness and increased credibility of the nurses with other professionals. The program provided an accurate evaluation of each staff member's current performance level, specific learning needs, and potential for working in alternate patient settings. It also allowed for professional recognition of individual staff members. These findings have been validated by Robinson and Barberis-Ryan (1995) in the implementation of a house-wide program at an acute care facility in New York.

The Competency Achievement Program (CAP) at Braddock General Hospital (Benedum, Kalup, & Freed, 1990) is a comprehensive plan which links orientation and ongoing continuing education through annual staff competency assessment. The developers of this program identified four criteria which were essential to success:

* administrative support and commitment,
* inclusion of managers and supervisors at all levels of program development,
* methods to overcome resistance to evaluation, and
* ongoing program revision.

The competency assessment program at Mercy Medical Center is structured as the initial component of the performance appraisal process. Although beyond the scope of this book, the other components of performance appraisal include the evaluation of consistency, proficiency, and achievement. We have defined competency as *the ability to perform basic job responsibilities* rather than as proficiency as other programs have used the term.

Competency assessment in our facility is a PASS/FAIL measure of job performance which occurs prior to evaluating how consistently (proficiently) the individual performs. We employ Alspach's definition of motor, attitudinal, and cognitive abilities to identify individual competencies. Only the essential characteristics of abilities define the performance standards against which each employee is evaluated. Although we employ Alspach's definition (1993) of motor, attitudinal, and cognitive abilities to identify individual competencies, most of our competencies remain in the realm of motor skills at this time. Each year as we review the program, we are encouraging departments to add more attitudinal and cognitive abilities to their plans. The focus of this manual is to provide competency assessment tools and the guidelines for development of a multidisciplinary program.

REFERENCES

Alspach, G. (May, 1993). *Competency-Based Orientation.* Presented at Nursing Staff Development 1993, Washington, DC.

Benedum, E., Kalup, M., Freed, D.; (1990), "A Competency Achievement Program for Direct Caregivers." *Nursing Management.* 21(5), 32-35.

Benner, P. (1982). "Issues in Competency-Based Testing." *Nursing Outlook.* 30(5), 303-309.

del Bueno, D.J., (May, 1994). *Competency based: Focus on Outcomes* presented at Medical College of Pennsylvania/NNSDO Nursing Staff Development & Management '94, Washington, DC.

del Bueno, D.J.,; Altano, R.; (1984). "Competency-Based Education: No Magic Feather." *Nursing Management.* 15(4), 48-53.

del Bueno, D. J., Werks, L.& Brown-Stewart, P. (1987). "Clinical Assessment Centers: A Cost-Effective Alternative for Competency Development." *Nursing Economics.* 5(1), 21-26.

DiMauro, K & Mack, L.B. (1989). "A Competency-Based Orientation Program for the Clinical Nurse Specialist,." *Journal of Continuing Education In Nursing.* 20(2), 74-78.

Glotz, N., Johnsen, G.& Johnson, R. (1994). "Advancing Clinical Excellence: Competency-Based Patient Care. *Nursing Management.* 25(1), 42-44.

1995 Accreditation Manual for Hospitals. Volume 1: Standards. (1994). Joint Commission on Accreditation of Healthcare Organizations. Oakbrook Terrace, IL.

Kemp, J. (1985). *The Instructional Design Process.* Harper & Row: New York, NY.

Lawinger, S.J. (1991). "Competency-Based Orientation Program for a Surgical Intensive Therapy Unit." *Critical Care Nurse.* 11(4), 36-44.

Morgan, M.K., Irby, D. (1978). *Evaluating Clinical Competency in the Health Professions.* The C.V. Mosbey Company: St. Louis, MO.

O'Grady, T & O'Brien, A. (1992). "A guide to Competency-Based Orientation: Develop Your Own Program." *Journal of Staff Development.* 8(3), 128-133.

Peterson, K.J. (1991). "Competency-Based Orientation Program for a Cardiovascular Surgery Unit," *Critical Care Nurse.* 11(2), 32-33.

Redus, K.M. (1994). "A Literature Review of Competency-Based Orientation for Nurses. *Journal of Nursing Staff Development.* 10(5), 239-243.

Robinson, S.M. & Barberis-Ryan, C. (1995). "Competency Assessment: A Systematic Approach." *Nursing Management.* 26(2), 40-44.

References Continued:

Schmaus, D. (1987). "Competency-Based Education: Its Implication In the OR. *AORN Journal*. 45(2), 474-482.

Selfridge, J. (1984). "A Competency-Based Orientation for the Emergency Department." *Journal of Emergency Nursing*. 10(5), 246-253.

Stewart, S.L.& Vitello-Cicciu, J.M. (1989). "Defining a Competency-Based Orientation Program for the Care of Cardiac Surgical Patients." *Journal of Cardiovascular Nursing*. 3(3), 34-41.

Trautman, D.& Watson, J.E. (1995). "Implementing Continued Clinical Competency Evaluation in the Emergency Department." *Journal of Staff Development*. 11(1), 41-47.

CHAPTER 2

DEVELOPMENT OF A COMPETENCY PROGRAM

Chapter 2

DEVELOPMENT OF A COMPETENCY PROGRAM

Establishment of the General Policy

The initial step in developing a Competency Assessment program is to establish the general policy governing the program and the procedures which will guide it. A small committee of 3-6 members is adequate to develop the policy draft. At minimum, committee membership needs to include representation from Human Resources, Staff Development, and the different departments participating in the program.

Although each institution's policy will be influenced by its mission and employee relations policies, there are several components which will be common to most institutions. The policy needs to define:

* which employees will be required to participate,
* the frequency of testing, and
* the consequences of failure.

Additional components which improve the policy's strength include definitions of competence, a description of who the evaluators will be, and a description of the consequences of avoidance of testing. Figure 1 shows an example of the current policy and procedures established for competency assessment at Mercy Medical Center in Baltimore, Maryland.

Figure 1: Policy For Staff Competency Assessment

Purpose:

To assure that all patient care providers are competent to perform assigned responsibilities in their specific areas of clinical practice.

Policy:

All staff members will meet their role-specific-competencies as outlined in their job performance standards. Failure to meet competency standards may result in termination as outlined below.

Procedure:

Staff will be assessed for ongoing competence at the following time intervals:

1. At time of employment, competence will be established by educational background, licensure/certification, and previous experience/references. Written tests may be required for certain positions.

2. During orientation, each staff member will complete a department-specific Performance Evaluation Tool (skills checklist/critical behaviors checklist). It is also expected that each new hire complete the specific competency assessments required on an on-going basis of the job description.

3. In addition to the annual OSHA-mandated testing and other regulatory requirements such as CPR, each staff member in the Patient Care Services Department is responsible for completing their role-specific competency assessment annually.

Key Points

1. Completion of mandatory inservices will be validated by the Manager or their designee utilizing the Meditech Credentialing Database.

2. The initial testing period for competencies is established by departmental policy. The disciplinary process will be initiated for staff members who fail to comply with the testing plan at the conclusion of the original testing period.

3. Staff members are provided a total of two opportunities to successfully complete competency testing. All (100%) of the Performance Criteria must be completed appropriately in order

to achieve successful testing.

Staff members who fail to adequately complete any competency are not to perform those skills until they have successfully passed retesting. Remediation and retesting will be provided by the Manager (or designee) within two weeks of the initial testing period. Staff who are unable to successfully complete competency at the second testing will be referred to Human Resources for counseling regarding vacant positions for which they may be qualified.

4. Any staff member who is not initially successful with any component of any specific competency, and has a history of failing the same competency in the previous year, will be tested on the entire competency on a quarterly basis for 3 successive quarters by the Manager or designee.

   Staff who experience a subsequent quarterly failure or fail the next annual testing of that same competency will not be given further remediation. They will be referred to Human Resources for counseling regarding vacant positions for which they may be qualified.

5. Staff who have been referred to Human Resources for inadequately meeting role-specific competency standards will have one month to transfer to another position for which they are qualified. Since the Medical Center cannot maintain staff in unbudgeted positions, staff who have not transferred after one month will be terminated from employment.

   Should termination of employment become necessary under the above conditions, the employee will be eligible for rehire into an unfilled budgeted position for which they qualify. The employee can be rehired with the same level of benefits and seniority for up to 3 months after their termination. Their new salary will be based on the target market for the new position.

6. This policy does not supersede the Internal Transfer Policy.

Components of the Policy

I. How is competence defined?

The general policy for the institution needs to describe how successful completion of competency testing will be *operationally defined.* As shown in Figure 1 - Key Point 3, Mercy Medical Center operationalized successful testing as "appropriately completing 100% of the performance criteria." With this operational definition and with competencies which are Pass/Fail in nature, the performance standards identified on the evaluation tools should contain only those criteria that are critical to safe performance of the behavior.

II. Which employees are included?

Although staff competence has been a concern of the Joint Commission on Accreditation of Healthcare Organizations (JCAHO) since 1980, a standard which required a mechanism for ongoing evaluation of individual staff competence was not required until 1991, when it was established for nurses. In 1995, the Joint Commission will require institutions to implement a mechanism for assessing individual competence of all direct care providers (JCAHO Conference, "Joint Commission Standards for Nursing Care," Harrisburg, Pennsylvania, March, 1994). In 1996, the requirement will be extended to all hospital employees in all departments (JCAHO Conference, "An Executive Briefing for Hospital Leadership," Baltimore, Maryland, September, 1994).

III. Who should assess competence?

The general policy should describe who will assess the competency of staff members. Most competency assessment programs are based on the premise that competence is tested by a recognized or certified expert in the field or skill, such as Clinical Nurse Specialists or Senior Medical Technicians. A similar method, often used in large departments, is called "Train the Trainer," in which the acknowledged expert tests and accredits a few other competent employees. These second-level experts then join the original trainer in testing other staff members. In contrast, small, highly specialized departments may need to collaborate with colleagues in similar departments or in other institutions to complete the assessment process. Another way to assess competence is through peer or self-review; however, this requires sets of performance criteria which contain absolute delineation's of the standards and a clear sense of staff integrity.

IV. How frequently should competence be tested?

A. Prior to employment

Prior to employment, competence is established through previous experience, credentials, references, and education. However, these components do not necessarily measure an individual's ability to perform up to expectations. Pre-employment screenings such as typing tests are an example of true competency testing prior to employment. Share days, in which prospective employees work with current staff members, may also generate pre-employment knowledge of competence.

B. During orientation

Historically, the purpose of orientation to a new job has been to familiarize the new employee with the specific institution and department in which they have been hired. A competency-based orientation is built upon measurable objectives which allow for evaluation of individual competence and for individual adjustments in the length and scope of the orientation based on prior abilities and experiences (O'Grady & O'Brien, 1992). The new Joint Commission standards (1995) state that all department-specific orientations should include an evaluation of competence. All high volume skills should be addressed during orientation Additionally, all relevant patient care and electrical equipment must be included according to the 1995 JCAHO orientation and plant safety standards - see Figure 2, #8 for examples.

At Mercy, we require a Clinical Performance Tool (such as Figure 2) to be completed on all employees during orientation (see Figure 1, Procedure 2). This tool helps evaluate how a broad spectrum of the performance criteria and/or sub-objectives outlined in the orientation and job performance standards is measured. We require that all competencies on the annual on-going competency assessment be included in this tool. This evaluation of competence validates references to individual competence from previous employers and must be completed on all employees regardless of previous experience. Individuals who are unable to completently perform the abilities identified within the orientation timeline are redeployed or terminated.

Patient Care Services Department

CLINICAL PERFORMANCE EVALUATION: CLERICAL ASSOCIATE

NAME	To be Completed by Orientee		To be Completed by Preceptor		COMMENTS
	HAVE HAD EXPERIENCE- FEEL COMFORTABLE DOING	LIMITED EXPERIENCE ASSISTANCE NEEDED	DEMONSTRATED WITH ASSISTANCE	MANAGED INDEPENDENTLY	
COMMUNICATION					
1. Communicates effectively with healthcare team					
2. Maintains the patient/family rights to privacy and confidentiality.					
3. Appropriately accesses chain of command for patient/family.					
DOCUMENTATION					
1. Correctely utilizes abbrefiations used by medical and nursing staff.					
2. Correctly documents all graphic data (weights, vital signs, etc.)					
3. Prepares charts for admission, discharge, transfer, death.					
4. Maintains Kardex/Carepaths appropriately.					
5. Utilizes medication/treatment schedules appropriately.					
6. Performs char checks, according to unit policy.					
7. Maintains Medex correctly.					

13

NAME	To be Completed by Orientee			To be Completed by Preceptor		COMMENTS
	HAVE HAD EXPERIENCE FEEL COMFORTABLE DOING	LIMITED EXPERIENCE ASSISTANCE NEEDED	DEMONSTRATED WITH ASSISTANCE	MANAGED INDEPENDENTLY		
8. Correctly uses Meditech System						
Order Entry						
PCI						
Materials Management						
Dietary						
Charge Entry						
9. Checks OR preparation.						
MAINTAINS A SAFE AND CLEAN ENVIRONMENT						
1. Checks emergency equipment.						
2. Performs Blood Glucose Monitoring Controls procedure.						
3. Checks and replaces stock medications.						
4. Participates in environmental rounds.						
PERSONAL DEVELOPMENT						
1. Demonstrates adherence to hospital policy and procedure.						

Recommendations:

Items the Clerical Associate will need further assistance with are:

PRECEPTOR: _____

ORIENTEE: _____

NURSE MANAGER/DESIGNATE: _____

14

C. Ongoing Assessment

After new employees have completed orientation, individual competence should be assessed at defined intervals throughout an employee's tenure. Each institution or department must identify what the defined intervals will be for their own staff. Additionally, various federal and state regulating agencies (e.g. OSHA, CLIA '88) or certifying agencies (e.g. State Boards for professional practice) may dictate the frequency of testing for specific competencies. Although there is no definitive statement for required frequency of testing, annual competency testing as a part of the performance appraisal process is quite common among those institutions who have already developed ongoing competency assessment programs (Benedum, Kalup, & Freed, 1990; Glotz, Johnsen, & Johnson, 1995; Robinson & Barberis-Ryan, 1995; Trautman & Watson, 1995).

V. What happens to staff who fail or avoid testing?

A critical component of the competency assessment policy is the clear delineation of the consequences of failure or avoidance of testing. Failure may necessitate remediation, retesting, or re-employment (refer to Key Points 3-5 of Figure 1). An employee who is unsuccessful in meeting performance criteria of a competency should not be performing that specific duty until successful retesting is completed. The policy should describe the parameters of remediation, including how long and how many times it will be offered. It is important that retesting occur quickly so that employees may resume the full work assignments expected of their position. The policy should also address the issue of re-employment/transfer to another department or termination if remediation is unsuccessful. It is critical to include the Human Resource Department of the institution in this discussion. The consequences of avoidance of testing also need to be addressed in general policy (Figure 1 - Key Point 2). Because disciplinary action may need to be taken, it is imperative that avoidance be defined concretely and that the policy be explained to each employee.

Development of Departmental Competency Assessment Plans

The second step in creating a competency assessment program is to develop department-specific plans. These plans identify the specific competencies (only a representative sample of the broad list utilized in orientation is necessary) which will be assessed for each job position during the ongoing component of competency assessment, list performance criteria which will define successful completion of the testing for each competency, and describe the testing process. Although the actual performance criteria of a specific competency may be revised due to changes in policy, technology, research findings, or new regulations, and additional competencies may be added for a variety of needs, individual JCAHO surveyors have shown a desire to see that each competency originally identified in the plan remains on the plan for the three year cycle between JCAHO visits. The exact number of competencies identified on the plan will depend on the scope of practice of the position. The methods of testing chosen by a department may be based on the available resources within the department, the experience available, and the type of competency.

I. Which skills should be included for ongoing assessment?

Because they are experts in the daily routines and expectations of their job, it is imperative that staff members participate in the selection of skills to be included in the plan. Due to the extensive time resources needed to evaluate competency, the identified competencies in the ongoing program may be a sub-set of behaviors found on the orientation performance evaluation tool, mentioned earlier, for that job position. Figure 3 provides an example of the skills chosen by the nursing staff in an Emergency Department for their competency assessment plan. As shown, the plan should identify a unique set of competencies for each job position in the department, although similar competencies may overlap for different levels of staff. It is not necessary for every department and every position to have the same number of skills identified in their plans. Note the difference between the Registered Nurse and ED Technician positions in figure 3. In contrast to the high volume behaviors evaluated during orientation, the skills identified in the ongoing competency assessment plans should meet at least one of the following criteria:

* High Risk (physically, emotionally, or legally to patient, employee, or the institution), (see Figure 3, #1 of the RN list)
* Life-threatening (see Figure 3, #2 of the RN list)

* Problem prone (see Figure 3, #2 of the RN list, and/or
* Low volume (done less than weekly) (see Figure 3, #5 of the ED Technician list)

   Most psychomotor skills can be included easily in competency assessment programsusing actual clinical situations or laboratory simulations. Although more difficult to measure and remediate, cognitive skills such as delegating work assignments, interpretation of diagnostic tests, recognition of abuse, or prioritization of house-wide respiratory therapy are required criteria as well. These competencies may be assessed by direct observation, documentation of patient needs, or written examinations. Skills and topics which are not measured easily (such as ethical decision making) or cannot be evaluated through clinical simulation (such as management of precipitous birth/BOA in the Emergency Department, Figure 3, Educational Activity #2) may still be included in the program through the use of educational activities. These activities are no less important than the other topics; they are just presented in a different methodology. A list of educational activities is not currently required by the regulatory agencies.

Figure 3: Sample Department Plan

Policy/Procedure/Protocol:
Competency Assessment Plan for Emergency Department

Distribution:
Unit-Specific

Purpose:
To assure that all nursing staff members in the ED meet the identified competencies established for their job description.

Policy:
The following competencies/educational activities will be assessed annually for each staff member:

REGISTERED NURSES

Competency Assessments
1. Equipment set-up and maintenance for arterial line monitoring
2. Defibrillation
3. ABG collection
4. Glucose monitoring
5. Nursing assessment (every 2 years)
6. Delegating work assignments

Educational Activities
1. Review the utilization of ventilators
2. Review the care of the family with a precipitous birth/BOA
3. Review the function of internal and external pacemakers
4. Review pediatric cardiac arrest management
5. Review of chest tube set-up and management

ED TECHNICIANS

Competency Assessments
1. 1. EKG lead application
2. Cardiac monitor application
3. Peripheral venipuncture
4. Taking vital signs
5. Glucose monitoring

II. How are the Performance Criteria established?

After the specific competencies have been identified, the performance criteria, against which successful competency testing is measured, must be established. These criteria can be garnered from policy and procedure manuals, published Professional Standards, current textbooks, and interviews with staff who complete the task daily. The performance criteria do not necessarily need to include **every** step found in a procedure but **MUST** include those critical behaviors which define competence or safety. Figure 4 presents the eight performance criteria identified for the competency of Autovac Preparation. As seen in this competency tool, each criteria should be written with one action verb and in such a way that clearly notes whether the employee included this step in the performance of the competency.

In order to ensure reliable testing results, staff members **must** be involved in validating all performance criteria before the tools are placed into service. There should only be one set of criteria for any particular competency. Multiple departments which identify the same competency need to collaborate in developing the performance criteria. The criteria then need to be validated by staff members in each department, especially if they have not been involved in the development of the plans or criteria. On the occasion that more than one set of criteria is developed for the same competency by various departments, different titles should be given to each set, with differences justified in writing.

Patient Care Services

NAME _____
UNIT _____
DATE _____

COMPETENCY: Autovac Preparation		
PERFORMANCE CRITERIA	**COMPLETED BY STAFF**	
1. Maintains sterile technique during transfer of tubing and canister for circulator.	Y	N
2. Removes trocar cover safely.	Y	N
3. Safely passes trocar with drainage tubing to surgeon.	Y	N
4. Retrieves trocar safely.	Y	N
5. Places trocar in needle counter.	Y	N
6. Injects anticoagulant into autovac canister, using the appropriate port as ordered.	Y	N
7. Marks designated area on canister with date, time of institution and amount of additive.	Y	N
8. Disposes trocar, according to unit standards.	Y	N
COMMENTS:		

autovac.94

Evaluator_____

III. How is the methodology for testing chosen?

Staff members need a clear understanding of the method and timing of all competency testing. This information should be presented in departmental orientation and updated when applicable.

The method of testing for competence depends on the type of skill to be evaluated, the potential risk to those involved, and the available resources. Competence in most psychomotor skills can be assessed during actual care situations sunless the risk to the patient is too great or there are other ethical or confidential dilemmas. For example, CPR is always tested with mannequins because of the risk to the "victim," while fetal monitoring or EKG rhythm is typically tested with old strips so that the employee may concentrate on making accurate clinical judgements based on the interpretations during real-life emergency situations without fearing the testing component. Clinical simulations such as mock codes can be a viable alternative to direct observation of practice. One excellent method of testing and reviewing skills with staff members is to videotape their behavior and allow the staff to evaluate their own performance. Case study interpretation, computer-assisted instruction, interactive video, and certain types of documentation such as patient assignments, diet histories, and care plans may also suffice to demonstrate competency for cognitive skills.

Each department should establish and publicize when staff members are to be assessed. Small departments with limited resources may wish to test all employees on a specific competency each month. One effective strategy is to utilize a "competency marathon" in which multiple staff members are tested, usually for psychomotor skills, in a clinical situation. Larger departments may choose to test each employee on all competencies during their anniversary month of employment. Regardless of the department's choice, it is essential that employees understand their personal responsibility in the testing process to eliminate avoidance. Department managers may need to increase the number of on-duty staff during massive competency testing periods to ensure that staffing levels are adequate and that patient care is not compromised.

Monitoring Compliance

The final step in developing a Competency Assessment program is to identify how compliance will be monitored and evaluated. Compliance reports must be maintained for the three-year cycles between JCAHO surveys; however, other regulatory agencies may require that such information be kept longer. The JCAHO requires that each department maintain the records of their own personnel and than an annual competency compliance report be sent to the governing board. At Mercy Medical Center, each department maintains a department summary (see Figure 5) which is forwarded monthly to Administration and annually to the central staff development department for inclusion in the agency-wide compliance report. In other institutions, the central department may be the Human Resource Department or Risk Management Department depending on the institution's organizational structure.

Date of Competency Attainment

Unit: _____   Year: _____   Positions: _____

Staff Member	Blood Born Pathogens	Hazardous Waste	Fire & Safety	TB	Gloucose Monitoring	CPR	Defibrillation	ABG Collection

CHAPTER 3

DEPARTMENT-SPECIFIC PLANS

Chapter 3

DEPARTMENT-SPECIFIC PLANS

Outlines of the competency plans developed by the Patient Care Department within a general community hospital are provided. These outlines include those competencies that were deemed to be appropriate for the unit/department.

Each plan includes the distribution, purpose, policy, and staff members involved in the plan. The competencies and/or educational activities for each staff member are identified. The specific plan for the Pathology Department varies slightly from the format of the other plans due to necessary compliance with CLIA'88.

The plan(s) may need to be individualized by each facility, based on the scope of services provided and the staff mix in the unit/department. It is recommended that the department-specific plans be reviewed on an annual basis and additionally whenever there is a significant change in the roles and responsibilities of the staff.

Chapter Contents

Ambulatory Services
> Medical Clinic
>> RN
>> Nursing Assistant
> OB/GYN Clinic
>> RN
>> Nursing Assistant
> Pre-Admission Testing (PAT)
>> Nurse Practitioner
>> PAT Coordinator
>> Registrar/Tech/Radiology Tech

Critical Care Nursing
> Critical Care Unit
>> RN
>> Critical Care Technician
>> EMT/P Technician
> Progressive Care Unit
>> RN
>> Nursing Technician
>> Nursing Assistant
>> Monitor Technician

Emergency Department
> RN
> ED Technicians

Heart Center
> EKG Technician
> Cardiology Tech I
> Cardiology Tech II
> Echocardiographer
> Cardiac Catherterization Technologist
> Cardiac Catherterization RN

IV Therapy Department
> RN
> IV Therapy Technician

Medical-Surgical Nursing

<u>Medical-Surgical Unit</u>
- RN
- LPN
- Nursing Technician
- Nursing Assistant
- Clerical Associates

<u>Orthopedic Unit</u>
- RN
- LPN
- Nursing Technician
- Nursing Assistants
- Clerical Associates

<u>Women's Unit</u>
- RN
- LPN
- Nursing Technician
- Nursing Assistant
- Clerical Associates
- Unit Clerk/Transportation Technician

Nuclear Medicine Department
- Senior Technologist
- Nuclear Medicine Technologist

Nutrition and Food Services
- Clinical Dietitians
- Dietetic Technicians
- Nutrition Service Representatives

Occupational Therapy Department
- Registered Occupational Therapist
- Certified Occupational Therapy Assistant

Oncology Nursing

<u>Oncology Unit</u>
- RN
- LPN
- Nursing Technician
- Nursing Assistant

<u>Outpatient Chemotherapy</u>
- RN

Pastoral Care Department
    Chaplain

Pathology Department

Pediatric Nursing
    <u>Pediatric Unit (Inpatient)</u>
        RN
        Nursing Technician
        Nursing Assistant
    <u>Pediatric Clinic</u>
        RN
        Nursing Assistant

Perinatal Nursing
    <u>Antepartal Diagnostic Center</u>
        RN
        Nursing Technician
    <u>Labor and Delivery</u>
        RN
        Nursing Technician
    <u>Mother-Baby</u>
        RN
        LPN
        Nursing Technician
        Nursing Assistant
    <u>NICU</u>
        RN

Psychiatric/Mental Health Services
    <u>Chemical Dependency Unit</u>
        RN
        Nursing Assistant
    <u>Eating Disorders Unit</u>
        RN

Radiology Department
        Technologists
        Angio/Cardiac Cath Technologist
        CT Technologist
        MRI Technologist
        Ultrasound Technologist

Rehabilitation Medicine Department
        Physical Therapist
        Physical Therapist Assistant
        Physical Therapy Aid

Respiratory Care Department
        Respiratory Care Practitioner

Speech Language Pathology Department
        Speech/Language Pathologist

Staff Development
        Clinical Educator
        Professional Development Coordinator
        Educational Support Specialist

Surgical Services
        <u>Endoscopy</u>
                RN
                Technician
        <u>Operating Room</u>
                RN
                Nursing Technician
                Surgical Technician
                Sterile Supply Technician
                OR Transporter
        <u>Pre-Operative Ambulatory Surgery</u>
                RN
                Nursing Technician
                Nursing Assistant
        <u>Post Anesthesia Care Unit (PACU)</u>
                RN
                Nursing Technician
        <u>Post-Operative Ambulatory Surgery</u>
                RN
                Nursing Technician

AMBULATORY SERVICES

POLICY/PROCEDURE/PROTOCOL:
Competency Assessment Plan for Medical Clinic

DISTRIBUTION:
Unit-Specific

PURPOSE:
To assure that all nursing staff members in the Medical Clinic meet the identified competencies established for their job description.

POLICY:
The following competencies/educational activities will be assessed annually for each staff member:

REGISTERED NURSE
Competency Assessments
1. Providing Diabetic Teaching
2. Teaching Injection Techniques
3. IV Discontinuation
4. Glucose Monitoring
5. Nursing Assessment (every 2 years)
6. Delegating Work Assignments

NURSING ASSISTANT
Competency Assessments
1. Taking Vital Signs
2. Assisting with Medical Clinic Procedures
3. Collecting a Clean Catch Urine Specimen

AMBULATORY SERVICES

POLICY/PROCEDURE/PROTOCOL:
Competency Assessment Plan for OB/GYN Clinic

DISTRIBUTION:
Unit-Specific

PURPOSE:
To assure that all nursing staff members in the OB/GYN Clinic meet the identified competencies established for their job description.

POLICY:
The following competencies/educational activities will be assessed annually for each staff member:

REGISTERED NURSE
Competency Assessments
1. Verification of Pregnancy
2. Nursing Assessment of the Ambulatory OB Client
3. STD Treatment
4. Glucose Monitoring
5. Nursing Assessment (every 2 years)
6. Delegating Work Assignments

NURSING ASSISTANT
Competency Assessments
1. Assist With Cervical Specimens
2. Set-Up Patient for Pelvic Exam
3. Testing Urine

AMBULATORY SERVICES

POLICY/PROCEDURE/PROTOCOL:
Competency Assessment Plan for Pre-Admission Testing (PAT)

DISTRIBUTION:
Department-Wide

PURPOSE:
To assure that all staff members in Pre-Admission Testing (PAT) meet the identified competence established for their job description.

POLICY:
The following competencies/educational activities will be assessed annually for each staff member:

NURSE PRACTITIONER
Competency Assessments
1. ECG Interpretation

Educational Activities
1. Providing Diabetic Teaching
3. Hypertensive/Cardiac Preventive Teaching

PAT COORDINATOR
Competency Assessments
1. Peripheral Venipuncture for Blood Specimens
2. Obtaining a 12 Lead EKG
3. Collecting a Clean-Catch Urine Specimen

REGISTRAR/TECH/RADIOLOGY TECH
Competency Assessments
1. Peripheral Venipuncture for Blood Specimens
2. Obtaining a 12 Lead EKG
3. Collecting a Clean Catch Urine Specimen

CRITICAL CARE

POLICY/PROCEDURE/PROTOCOL:
Competency Assessment Plan for Critical Care Unit

DISTRIBUTION:
Unit-Specific

PURPOSE:
To assure that all nursing staff members in the CCU meet the identified competencies established for their job description.

POLICY:
The following competencies/educational activities will be assessed annually for each staff member:

REGISTERED NURSE
Competency Assessments
1. ABG Collection
2. Defibrillation
3. Thermodilution Catheters
4. Glucose Monitoring
5. Nursing Assessment (every 2 years)
6. Delegating Work Assignments

Educational Activities
1. Review of Emergency Cardiac Drugs
2. Review of Anesthesia Drugs/Reversal Drugs

CRITICAL CARE TECHNICIAN
Competency Assessments
1. Obtain EKG
2. Taking Vital Signs
3. Glucose Monitoring
4. ET or Tracheal Suctioning
5. Foley Catheter Insertion
6. NG Insertion

EMT/P TECHNICIAN
Competency Assessments
1. Peripheral Venipuncture
2. Glucose Monitoring

CRITICAL CARE

POLICY/PROCEDURE/PROTOCOL:
Competency Assessment Plan for Progressive Care Unit

DISTRIBUTION:
Unit-Specific

PURPOSE:
To assure that all staff members of the Progressive Care Unit meet the identified competencies established for their job description.

POLICY:
The following competencies/educational activities will be assessed annually for each staff member:

REGISTERED NURSE
Competency Assessments
1. Defibrillation
2. Interpretation of Arrthythmias (written test)
3. Emergency Drug Administration (written test)
4. Glucose Monitoring
5. Nursing Assessment (every 2 years)
6. Delegating Work Assignments

NURSING TECHNICIAN
Competency Assessments
1. Prepare Equipment for Oxygen Administration
2. Obtain a 12 Lead EKG
3. Apply Telemetry Leads
4. Taking Vital Signs
5. Glucose Monitoring

NURSING ASSISTANT
Competency Assessments
1. Chart I&O
2. Apply Telemetry Leads
3. Prepare Equipment for Oxygen Administration
4. Taking Vital Signs

CRITICAL CARE
MONITOR TECHNICIANS
Competency Assessments

1. Recognize Selected Arrhythmia (written test)
2. Apply Telemetry Leads

EMERGENCY DEPARTMENT

POLICY/PROCEDURE/PROTOCOL:
Competency Assessment Plan for Emergency Department

DISTRIBUTION:
Department-Wide

PURPOSE:
To assure that all nursing staff members in the Emergency Department meet the identified competencies established for their job description.

POLICY:
The following competencies/educational activities will be assessed **annually** for each staff member:

REGISTERED NURSE
Competency Assessments
1. Equipment Set-Up and Maintenance for Arterial Line Monitoring
2. Defibrillation
3. ABG Collection
4. Glucose Monitoring
5. Nursing Assessment (every 2 years)
6. Delegating Work Assignments

Educational Activities
1. Review the Utilization of Ventilators
2. Review the Care of the Family With a Precipitous Birth/BOA
3. Review the Function of Internal and External Pacemakers
4. Review of Pediatric Cardiac Arrest Management
5. Review of Chest Tube Set-Up and Management

EMERGENCY DEPARTMENT TECHNICIAN
Competency Assessments
1. EKG Lead Application
2. Cardiac Monitor Application
3. Peripheral Venipuncture
4. Taking Vital Signs
5. Glucose Monitoring

HEART CENTER

POLICY/PROCEDURE/PROTOCOL:
Competency Assessment Plan for Heart Center

DISTRIBUTION:
Unit-Specific

PURPOSE:
To assure that all staff members in the Heart Center meet the identified competencies established for their job descriptions.

POLICY:
The following competencies/educational activities will be assessed annually for each staff member:

EKG TECHNICIAN
Competency Assessments:
1. Adult EKG
2. Pediatric EKG
3. Stress Test Procedures
4. Holter Monitor Application

CARDIOLOGY TECHNICIAN I
Competency Assessments:
1. Adult EKG
2. Adult/Pediatric Holter Monitoring
3. Stress Test Procedures

CARDIOLOGY TECHNICIAN II
Competency Assessments:
1. Adult EKG
2. Adult/Pediatric Holter Monitoring
3. Stress Test Procedures
4. Echocardiograms
5. Dopplers

ECHOCARDIOGRAPHER
Competency Assessments:
1. Adult Echocardiogram Procedures
2. Pediatric Echocardiogram Procedures
3. Doppler Procedures

CARDIAC CATHETERIZATION TECHNOLOGIST

Competency Assessments:
1. Venipuncture
2. Defibrillation
3. Scrubbing Procedures
4. Circulating Procedures

Educational Activities
1. Radiation Safety
2. Equipment Safety

CARDIAC CATHETERIZATION NURSE (RN)

Competency Assessments:
1. Venipuncture
2. IV Starts
3. Defibrillation
4. Cardiac Cath Circulating Procedures
5. Patient Assessment

Educational Activities:
1. Radiation Safety
2. Equipment Safety

ALL TECHNICAL AND NON-TECHNICAL STAFF

Educational Activities
1. CPR

IV THERAPY

POLICY/PROCEDURE/PROTOCOL:

Competency Assessment Plan for IV Therapy Department

DISTRIBUTION:

Department-Wide

PURPOSE:

To assure that all nursing staff members on the IV Team meet the identified competencies established for their job description.

POLICY:

The following competencies/educational activities will be assessed annually for each staff member:

REGISTERED NURSE

Competency Assessments

1. Central Line Access/Maintenance
2. Initiation of PCA Pumps
3. Implementation of Blood Transfusions
4. Initiation and Troubleshooting of Volumetric Infusion Pumps
5. Blood Collection from Central Lines

IV THERAPY TECHNICIAN

Competency Assessments

1. Obtain 12 Lead EKG
2. Peripheral Venipuncture for Blood Specimens

MEDICAL-SURGICAL NURSING

POLICY/PROCEDURE/PROTOCOL:
Competency Assessment Plan for General Medical/Surgical Unit

DISTRIBUTION:
All General Medical/Surgical Units

PURPOSE:
To assure that all nursing staff members on the General Medical/Surgical Units meet the identified competencies established for their job description.

POLICY:
The following competencies/educational activities will be assessed **annually** for each staff member:

REGISTERED NURSE
Competency Assessments
1. Chest Tube Management
2. Perform Trach Care
3. PCA Pump Maintenance
4. Administration of IV Push Medications
5. Perform Continuous Bladder Irrigations
6. Glucose Monitoring
7. Nursing Assessment (every 2 years)
8. Delegating Work Assignments

Educational Activities
1. Code Box Review

LICENSED PRACTICAL NURSE
Competency Assessments
1. Chest Tube Maintenance
2. Trach Care
3. Continuous Bladder Irrigation

Educational Activities
1. Code Box Review

NURSING TECHNICIAN
Competency Assessments
1. Application of EKG Leads
2. Insertion of Foley Catheter (M/F)
3. Oral/Pharyngeal Suctioning

4. Taking Vital Signs

<u>Educational Activities</u>
1. Review of Skin Integrity Changes During Healing
2. Review of Sterile Technique

NURSING ASSISTANT

<u>Competency Assessments</u>
1. Set-Up and Maintain Anti-Embolism Devices
2. Maintain Traction
3. Assist Patients with Feeding Techniques
4. Taking Vital Signs

CLERICAL ASSOCIATE

<u>Competency Assessments</u>
1. Computer Order Entry Skills (written test)
2. Medical Transcription (written test)

MEDICAL/SURGICAL NURSING

POLICY/PROCEDURE/PROTOCOL:
Competency Assessment Plan for Orthopedic Unit

DISTRIBUTION:
Unit-Specific

PURPOSE:
To assure that all nursing staff members on the Orthopedic Unit meet the identified competencies established for their job description.

POLICY:
The following competencies/educational activities will be assessed annually for each staff member:

REGISTERED NURSE
Competency Assessments
1. Maintenance of PCA Pump
2. Obtain EKG
3. Initiation and Maintenance of Selected Forms of Traction
4. Administer IV Push Medications
5. Glucose Monitoring
6. Nursing Assessment (every 2 years)
7. Delegating Work Assignments

Educational Activities
1. Code Box Review
2. Review of Trach Care

LICENSED PRACTICAL NURSE
Competency Assessments
1. Chest Tube Management
2. Obtain EKG
3. Traction: Initiation/Maintenance
4. Glucose Monitoring

Educational Activities
1. Code Box Review

NURSING TECHNICIAN
Competency Assessments
1. Apply EKG Leads
2. Insertion of Foley Catheters (M/F)

3. Tube Feeding
4. Taking Vital Signs
5. Glucose Monitoring

<u>Educational Activities</u>
1. Review Sterile Technique

NURSING ASSISTANT

<u>Competency Assessments</u>
1. Set-Up and Maintain Anti-Embolism Devices
2. Utilization of CPM Machine
3. Feeding Techniques
4. Taking Vital Signs

CLERICAL ASSOCIATE

<u>Competency Assessments</u>
1. Computer Order Entry (written test)
2. Medication Transcription (written test)

MEDICAL/SURGICAL NURSING

POLICY/PROCEDURE/PROTOCOL:
Competency Assessment Plan for Women's Service Unit

DISTRIBUTION:
Unit-Specific

PURPOSE:
To assure that all nursing staff members on the Women's Service Unit meet the identified competencies established for their job description.

POLICY:
The following competencies/educational activities will be assessed annually for each staff member:

REGISTERED NURSE
Competency Assessments
1. Management of Chest Tubes
2. PCA Maintenance
3. Obtain EKG
4. Administration of Selected IV Push Medications

Educational Activities
1. Review Code Box
2. Review of Community Support Services for Women

LICENSED PRACTICAL NURSE
Competency Assessments
1. Management of Chest Tubes
2. Obtain EKG

Educational Activities
1. Code Box Review
2. Review of Community Support Services for Women

NURSING TECHNICIAN
Competency Assessments
1. Application of EKG Leads
2. Insertion of Foley Catheters (M/F)
3. Implement Tube Feeding
4. Taking Vital Signs

Educational Activities
1. Review Sterile Technique

NURSING ASSISTANT

1. Application and Maintenance of Anti-Embolism Devices
2. Assisting Patients in Eating
3. Taking Vital Signs

UNIT CLERK/TRANSCRIPTION TECH
Competency Assessments

1. Utilization of Computer (Meditech) System
2. Charting Selected Graphic Data

NUCLEAR MEDICINE

POLICY/PROCEDURE/PROTOCOL:
Competency Assessment Plan for Nuclear Medicine

DISTRIBUTION:
Unit-Specific

PURPOSE:
To assure that all staff members in the Nuclear Medicine Department meet the identified competencies established for their job description.

POLICY:
The following competencies/educational activities will be assessed annually for each staff member:

SENIOR NUCLEAR MEDICINE TECHNOLOGIST
Competency Assessments
1. Manages Quality Control for the Department
2. Reviews Monthly Dosimeter Readings According to the ALARA Program
3. Performs a Bone Scan

Educational Activities
1. Radiation Safety
2. Camera Safety

NUCLEAR MEDICINE TECHNOLOGIST
Competency Assessments
1. Performing an Intrinsic Flood
2. Performing a Bone Scan According to Departmental Standards
3. Prepares, Calibrates and Administers Radiopharmaceuticals in an Aseptic Manner for Individual Scans Ordered Throughout the Day

Educational Activities
1. Radiation Safety
2. Camera Safety

NUTRITION AND FOOD SERVICES

POLICY/PROCEDURE/PROTOCOL:
Competency Assessment Plan for Nutrition Services

DISTRIBUTION:
Department-Wide

PURPOSE:
To assure that all Nutrition Service staff members meet the identified competencies established for their job description.

POLICY:
The following competencies/educational activities will be assessed **annually** for each staff member:

CLINICAL DIETITIAN (IN-PATIENT)
Competency Assessments
1. Nutritional Assessment of a Patient With a CVA
2. Nutritional Assessment of a Patient With Diabetes and Heart Disease
3. Medical Records Documentation
4. For NICU Dietitian Only, Nutritional Assessment of Pediatric Patient in a MVA

CLINICAL DIETITIAN (OUT-PATIENT)
Competency Assessments
1. Nutritional Assessment of a Patient with Gestational Diabetes
2. Nutritional Assessment of a Client Involved in Sports
3. Medical Record Documentation

DIETETIC TECHNICIAN
Competency Assessments
1. Screening and Leveling for Risk of Malnutrition
2. Correction of Diabetic Menus
3. Medical Record Documentation

NUTRITION SERVICE REPRESENTATIVE
<u>Competency Assessments</u>
1. Preparation of Menus for Distribution
2. Assisting Patients With Menu Selections
3. Ordering Special Food Items

OCCUPATIONAL THERAPY

POLICY/PROCEDURE/PROTOCOL:
Competency Assessment Plan for Occupational Therapy Department

DISTRIBUTION:
Unit-Specific

PURPOSE:
To assure that all Occupational Therapy staff members meet the identified competencies established for their job description.

POLICY:
The following competencies/educational activities will be assessed annually for each staff member.

REGISTERED OCCUPATIONAL THERAPIST/CERTIFIED OCCUPATIONAL THERAPY ASSISTANT

Competency Assessments
1. Application of Physical Agent Modalities
2. Application of Dynamic and Static Splinting
3. Screening/Evaluation and Treatment Process of Mastectomy Patients

Educational Activities
1. Attend an Accredited Continuing Education Course on the Use of Physical Agent Modalities
2. Attend/Present an Inservice on PAM/WC or Mastectomy Patients
3. Review Mastectomy Protocol
4. Review Literature on Advanced PAM

ONCOLOGY

POLICY/PROCEDURE/PROTOCOL:
Competency Assessment Plan for Oncology Unit

DISTRIBUTION:
Unit-Specific

PURPOSE:
To assure that all nursing staff members on the Oncology Unit meet the identified competencies established for their job description.

POLICY:
The following competencies/educational activities will be assessed annually for each staff member:

REGISTERED NURSE
Competency Assessments
1. Calculation of ANC
2. IV Site Assessment
3. Management of Chemotherapy Spill
4. PCA Initiation and Maintenance
5. Glucose Monitoring
6. Nursing Assessment (every 2 years)
7. Peripheral IV Insertion
8. Developing Work Assignments
Educational Activities
1. Review Code Cart/Code Response
2. Care of the Neutropenic/Thrombocytopenic Patient

LICENSED PRACTICAL NURSE
Competency Assessments
1. Management of Chemotherapy Spills
2. IV Site Assessment
3. Heme Urine and Stool Testing
4. Glucose Monitoring
Educational Activities
1. Care of the Neutropenic/Thrombocytopenic Patient

NURSING TECHNICIAN
Competency Assessments
1. Taking Vital Signs

2. Immediate Response to Chemotherapy Spills
3. Heme Urine and Stool Testing
4. Insertion of Foley Catheter
5. Glucose Monitoring

NURSING ASSISTANT
<u>Competency Assessments</u>
1. Collection/Testing of Urine and Stool Heme Specimens
2. Taking and Graphing Vital Signs
3. Immediate Response to Chemotherapy Spills

ONCOLOGY

POLICY/PROCEDURE/PROTOCOL:
Competency Assessment Plan for Outpatient Chemotherapy

DISTRIBUTION:
Unit-Specific

PURPOSE:
To assure that all nursing staff members on the Outpatient Chemotherapy
Unit meet the identified competencies established for their job description.

POLICY:
The following competencies/educational activities will be assessed **annually**
for each staff member:

REGISTERED NURSE
Competency Assessments
1. Peripheral IV Insertion and Maintenance
2. Accessing Central Lines
3. Interpretation of Selected Lab Values (written test)
4. Assessment of and Immediate Treatment for Extravasation
   of Chemotherapeutic Agents
5. Nursing Assessment (every 2 years)

PASTORAL CARE

POLICY/PROCEDURE/PROTOCOL:
Competency Assessment Plan for Pastoral Care

DISTRIBUTION:
Department-Wide

PURPOSE:
To assure that all Pastoral Care Chaplains meet the identified competencies established for their job description.

POLICY:
The following competencies/educational activities will be assessed annually for each staff member:

CHAPLAIN
Competency Assessments
1. Spiritual Assessment
2. Handwashing
3. Entering an Isolation Room

PATHOLOGY DEPARTMENT

POLICY/PROCEDURE/PROTOCOL:
Competency Assessment Plan for Pathology Department

DISTRIBUTION:
Department-Wide

PURPOSE:
To assure that all staff members in the Pathology Department meet the identified competencies established for their job description, according to CLIA '88. Compliance with CLIA '88 will consist of:

1. Direct Observation of Routine Patient Testing
2. Monitoring, Recording, and Reporting of Test Results by Review of the Database by the Technical Supervisors or Their Designee
3. Review of Intermediate Test Results or Worksheets, Quality Control Records, Proficiency Testing Results and Preventive Maintenance Records by the Technical Supervisors or Their Designee
4. Direct Observation of Performance of Instrument Maintenance and Function Checks
5. Assessment of Test Performance Accuracy Utilizing External Proficiency Testing
6. Assessment of Problem Solving Skills

POLICY:
The following competencies/educational activities will be assessed annually for each staff member:

Competency Assessments
1. Performing Selected Pathology Procedures
2. Performing Instrument Maintenance and Function Checks
3. Proficiency Testing of at Least 3 Analytes
4. Solving Problems in the Pathology Department

PEDIATRICS

POLICY/PROCEDURE/PROTOCOL:
Competency Assessment Plan for Inpatient Pediatric Unit

DISTRIBUTION:
Unit-Specific

PURPOSE:
To assure that all nursing staff members on the Pediatric Unit meet identified competencies established for their job description.

POLICY:
The following competencies/educational activities will be assessed annually for each staff member:

REGISTERED NURSE
Competency Assessments
1. Administration of IV Push Medications to Infants
2. Initiation and Maintenance of PCA Pump
3. Recognition of Abnormal Patterns on Cardio-Respiratory Monitors (written test)
4. Traction: Set-Up and Maintenance
5. Nursing Assessment (every 2 years)
6. Glucose Monitoring
7. Delegating Work Assignments

NURSING TECHNICIAN
Competency Assessments
1. Bottle Feeding Techniques
2. Set-Up IV Lines
3. Insertion of Foley Catheter (M/F)
4. Apply Cardiac-Apnea Monitor Leads
5. Taking Pediatric Vital Signs
6. Glucose Monitoring
Educational Activities
1. Review Pediatric Safety Issues

NURSING ASSISTANT
Competency Assessments
1. Bottle Feeding Techniques
2. Urine and Stool Testing

55

3. Taking Pediatric Vital Signs
<u>Educational Activities</u>
    1. Review of Pediatric Safety Issues

PEDIATRICS

POLICY/PROCEDURE/PROTOCOL:
Competency Assessment Plan for Pediatric Clinic

DISTRIBUTION:
Unit-Specific

PURPOSE:
To assure that all nursing staff members in the Pediatric Clinic meet the identified competencies established for their job description.

POLICY:
The following competencies/educational activities will be assessed annually for each staff member:

REGISTERED NURSE
Competency Assessments
1. Obtain EKG
2. Peripheral Venipuncture
3. Perform Audiometric Examination
4. Perform Peripheral IV Insertion
5. Perform Visual Screening Utilizing Titmus Tester
6. Nursing Assessment (every 2 years)
7. Glucose Monitoring

NURSING ASSISTANT
Competency Assessments
1. Taking Vital Signs
2. Utilization of Pediatric Scales

PERINATAL NURSING

POLICY/PROCEDURE/PROTOCOL:
Competency Assessment Plan for Antepartal Diagnostic Center

DISTRIBUTION:
Unit-Specific

PURPOSE:
To assure that all nursing staff members in the Antepartal Diagnostic Center meet the identified competencies established for their job description.

POLICY:
The following competencies/educational activities will be assessed annually for each staff member:

REGISTERED NURSE
Competency Assessments
1. Doing a Non Stress Test
2. Interpretation of Electronic Fetal Monitoring
3. Peripheral IV Insertion
4. Nursing Assessment (every 2 years)
5. Glucose Monitoring
6. Delegating Work Assignments

NURSING TECHNICIAN
Competency Assessments
1. Taking Vital Signs
2. Application of Electronic Fetal Monitoring Equipment
3. Glucose Monitoring

PERINATAL NURSING

POLICY/PROCEDURE/PROTOCOL:
Competency Assessment Plan for Labor and Delivery

DISTRIBUTION:
Unit-Specific

PURPOSE:
To assure that all nursing staff members in Labor and Delivery meet the identified competencies established for their job description.

POLICY:
The following competencies/educational activities will be assessed annually for each staff member:

REGISTERED NURSE
Competency Assessments
1. Interpretation of Electronic Fetal Monitoring Patterns
2. Initial Post-Delivery Newborn Assessment
3. Peripheral IV Insertion
4. Labor and Delivery Scrub Techniques
5. Perform Neonatal Resuscitation (every 2 years)
6. PCA Pump Set-Up
7. PCA Pump Maintenance
8. Glucose Monitoring
9. Nursing Assessment (every 2 years)
10. Delegating Work Assignments

Educational Activities
1. Management of Perinatal Loss support
2. Initiation of Breastfeeding
3. Amniotic Infusions

NURSING TECHNICIAN
Competency Assessments
1. Taking Vital Signs on Adults and Infants
2. Foley Catheter Insertion (M/F)
3. Application of Electronic Fetal Monitoring Equipment
4. Labor and Delivery Scrub Techniques
5. Glucose Monitoring

Educational Activities
1. Support for Newborn and Maternal Cardiac Arrests

PERINATAL NURSING

POLICY/PROCEDURE/PROTOCOL:
Competency Assessment Plan for Mother-Baby Unit

DISTRIBUTION:
Unit-Specific

PURPOSE:
To assure that all nursing staff members on the Mother-Baby Unit meet the identified competencies established for their job description.

POLICY:
The following competencies/educational activities will be assessed annually for each staff member:

REGISTERED NURSE
Competency Assessments
1. Interpretation of Electronic Fetal Monitoring
2. PCA Pump Initiation and Maintenance
3. Maternal Assessment
4. Newborn Assessment
5. PKU Draw
6. Breastfeeding Techniques
7. Managing Perinatal Loss
8. Nursing Assessment (every 2 years)
9. Glucose Monitoring
10. Delegating Work Assignments

LICENSED PRACTICAL NURSE
Competency Assessments
1. Application of Electronic Fetal Monitoring Equipment
2. Perinatal Loss
3. Recognition of Selected Abnormal Fetal Monitoring Patterns (written test)
4. PKU Draw
5. Management of Perinatal Loss support Program
6. Glucose Monitoring

NURSING TECHNICIAN
Competency Assessments
1. Maternal and Neonatal Vital Signs

2. PKU Draws
3. Apply External Fetal Monitoring Equipment
4. Obtain 30 Minute Electronic Fetal Monitoring Strip
5. Support for Family Experiencing Perinatal Loss
6. Glucose Monitoring

NURSING ASSISTANT
Competency Assessments
1. Take Maternal and Neonatal Vital Signs
2. Bottle Feeding Infants
3. Apply External Fetal Monitoring Equipment
4. Support of a Family After Perinatal Loss

PERINATAL NURSING

POLICY/PROCEDURE/PROTOCOL:
Competency Assessment Plan for Neonatal Intensive Care Unit

DISTRIBUTION:
Unit-Specific

PURPOSE:
To assure that all nursing staff members in the Neonatal Intensive Care Unit meet the identified competencies established for their job description.

POLICY:
The following competencies/educational activities will be assessed **annually** for each staff member:

REGISTERED NURSE
Competency Assessments
1. Perform Endotracheal Tube Suctioning
2. Set-Up and Maintain Chest tube
3. Assist with Exchange Transfusions
4. Perform Neonatal Resuscitation (every 2 years)
5. Neonatal Assessment

Educational Activities
1. Film Series on "Compromised Neonate"
2. Review Nursing Measures to Prevent IVH
3. Review of Management of Thermoregulation
4. Review Nursing Measures to Maintain Skin Integrity
5. Review Assessment of Parental Response to Having a Critically Ill Infant

PSYCHIATRIC/MENTAL HEALTH SERVICES

POLICY/PROCEDURE/PROTOCOL:
Competency Assessment Plan for Chemical Dependency Unit

DISTRIBUTION:
Unit-Specific

PURPOSE:
To assure that all nursing staff members on the Chemical Dependency Unit meet the identified competencies established for their job description.

POLICY:
The following competencies/educational activities will be assessed annually for each staff member:

REGISTERED NURSE
Competency Assessments
1. Administer IV Push Drugs
2. Peripheral Venipuncture
3. Glucose Monitoring
4. Nursing Assessment (every 2 years)
5. Delegating Work Assignments

Educational Activities
1. Code Box Review

NURSING ASSISTANT
Competency Assessments
1. Assembly of Chart Packs for Admission and Discharge
2. Charting Intake and Output
3. Taking vital Signs

PSYCHIATRIC/MENTAL HEALTH SERVICES

POLICY/PROCEDURE/PROTOCOL:
Competency Assessment Plan for Eating Disorders Unit

DISTRIBUTION:
Unit-Specific

PURPOSE:
To assure that all nursing staff members on the Eating Disorders Unit meet the identified competencies established for their job description.

POLICY:
The following competencies/educational activities will be assessed annually for each staff member:

REGISTERED NURSE
Competency Assessments
1. Assessment of Suicide Risk
2. Physical Assessment for Eating Disorder Danger Signs
3. Management of a Violent Patient
4. Glucose Monitoring
5. Nursing Assessment (every 2 years)

Educational Activities
1. Code Box Review
2. Review of Signs and Symptoms of Diabetic Complications
3. Review of Legal Issues of Restraint Use

RADIOLOGY

POLICY/PROCEDURE/PROTOCOL
Competency Assessment Plan for Radiology Department

DISTRIBUTION:
Department-Wide

PURPOSE:
To assure that all Radiology Department staff members meet the identified competencies established for their job description.

POLICY:
The following competencies/educational activities will be assessed **annually** for each staff member:

RADIOLOGY TECHNOLOGIST
Competency Assessments
1. Cervical Spine Exams
2. Verification/Documentation of Last Menstrual Period
3. Oxygen Management
4. Infusion Pump Management

ANGIO/CARDIAC CATH TECHNOLOGIST
Competency Assessments
1. Venipuncture
2. Defibrillation
3. Angio-Cardiac Cath Scrubbing
4. Angio-Cardiac Circulating

CT TECHNOLOGIST
Competency Assessments
1. Venipuncture
2. Biopsy/Drainage Procedures
3. Verification/Documentation of Blood Work Prior to Exam

MRI TECHNOLOGIST
Competency Assessments
1. Venipuncture
2. Carotid MRI Exams
3. Validation/Documentation of Patient's History

ULTRASOUND TECHNOLOGIST
<u>Competency Assessments</u>
1. Amniocentesis/Thoracentesis Procedures
2. Carotid Doppler Exams
3. Validation/Documentation of Patient's History

REHABILITATION MEDICINE

POLICY/PROCEDURE/PROTOCOL:

Competency Assessment Plan for Rehabilitation Medicine Department

DISTRIBUTION:

Department-Wide

PURPOSE:

To assure that all Physical Therapists in the Rehabilitation Medicine Department meet the identified competencies established for their job description.

POLICY:

The following competencies/educational activities will be assessed annually for each staff member:

PHYSICAL THERAPIST/PHYSICAL THERAPIST ASSISTANT

Competency Assessments
1. Computer Access (written test)
2. Deliver Ultrasound Therapy
3. Outpatient Documentation for Physical Therapy

PHYSICAL THERAPY AID

Competency Assessments
1. Dressing Change
2. Crutch Training
3. Whirlpool Cleansing

RESPIRATORY THERAPY

POLICY/PROCEDURE/PROTOCOL:
Competency Assessment Plan for Respiratory Care

DISTRIBUTION:
Department-Wide

PURPOSE:
To assure that all Respiratory Care staff members meet the identified competencies established for their job description.

POLICY:
The following competencies/educational activities will be assessed annually for each staff member.

RESPIRATORY CARE PRACTITIONER
Competency Assessments
1. Bronchial Hygiene
2. Oxygen Therapy
3. Arterial Blood Gas Sampling
4. Unit Rounds - CCU
5. Unit Rounds - NICU

SPEECH LANGUAGE PATHOLOGY

POLICY/PROCEDURE/PROTOCOL:
Competency Assessment Plan for Speech Language Pathologist

DISTRIBUTION:
Department-Wide

PURPOSE:
To assure that all Speech Pathologists in the Rehabilitation Department meet the identified competencies established for their job description.

POLICY:
The following competencies/educational activities will be assessed annually for each staff member:

SPEECH/LANGUAGE PATHOLOGIST
Competency Assessments
1. Modified Barium Swallow Study
2. Pediatric Screening Protocol
3. Discharge Report Dictation
4. Evaluation of CVA

Educational Activities
1. Review of Licensure for Speech Pathologists
2. Attend Mandatory Staff Inservices
3. Review of Therapy Materials

STAFF DEVELOPMENT

POLICY/PROCEDURE/PROTOCOL:

Competency Assessment Plan for Staff Development Department

DISTRIBUTION:

Department-Wide

PURPOSE:

To assure that all of the Staff Development Department members meet the identified competencies established for their job description.

POLICY:

The following competencies/educational activities will be assessed annually for each staff member.

PROFESSIONAL DEVELOPMENT COORDINATOR/ CLINICAL EDUCATOR

Competency Assessments
1. Oral Presentations to Adults
2. Coordination of Educational Program
3. Project Management Coordination Educational Activities

Educational Activities
1. CQI Update
2. JCAHO Update

EDUCATION SUPPORT SPECIALIST

Competency Assessments
1. Clerical support for Programs/Presentations
2. Use of Audi-visual Equipment
3. Use of Video Camera

Educational Activities
1. Computer Software Update

SURGICAL SERVICES

POLICY/PROCEDURE/PROTOCOL:
Competency Assessment Plan for Endoscopy

DISTRIBUTION:
Unit-Specific

PURPOSE:
To assure that all nursing staff members in Endoscopy meet the identified competencies established for their job description.

POLICY:
The following competencies/educational activities will be assessed annually for each staff member:

REGISTERED NURSE
Competency Assessment
1. Peripheral IV Insertion
2. Interpret Life-Threatening Arrhythmia's (written test)
3. Pre-Op Nursing Assessment
4. Nursing Assessment (every 2 years)
5. IV Conscious Sedation
6. Glucose Monitoring
7. Delegating Work Assignments

Educational Activities
1. Review of Anesthesia Drugs/Reversal Drugs
2. Review of Selected Cardiac Arrthymia Patterns

TECHNICIAN
Competency Assessments
1. Cleaning Scopes
2. Identification of ERCP Equipment

SURGICAL SERVICES

POLICY/PROCEDURE/PROTOCOL:
Competency Assessment Plan for the Operating Room

DISTRIBUTION:
Unit-Specific

PURPOSE:
To assure that all nursing staff members in the Operating Room will meet the identified competencies established for their job description.

POLICY:
The following competencies/educational activities will be assessed annually for each staff member:

REGISTERED NURSE
Competency Assessments
1. Circulating on Laparoscopic Cholecystectomy Procedures
2. Circulating on Laser Surgical Procedures
3. Circulating on Hysteroscopy
4. Midas Rex Set-Up and Clean-Up
5. Nursing Assessment (every 2 years)
6. Glucose Monitoring
7. Delegating Work Assignments

NURSING TECHNICIAN
Competency Assessments
1. Cleaning of Scopes
2. Utilization of Hall Power Equipment
3. Foley Catheter Insertion
4. Glucose Monitoring
5. Tourniquet Tank
6. Suction Hook-Up

SURGICAL TECHNICIAN
Competency Assessments
1. Scrubbing on Laparoscopic Cholecystectomy Procedures
2. Perform Sterile Technique
3. Utilization of Stackhouse Smoke Evacuator
4. Autovac Preparation
5. Maintenance of Suction During an Operative Procedure

STERILE SUPPLY TECHNICIAN
Competency Assessments
1. Operation and Challenging of Sterilizers
2. Patient Transport
3. Set-Up and Cleaning of Laproscopic Cholecystectomy Equipment
4. Cleaning Scopes
5. Harmonic Scalpel Cleaning

OPERATING ROOM TRANSPORTER
Competency Assessments
1. Patient Transport
2. Removal of Wastes
3. Disinfection
4. Maintenance of Gas Tank Gauges
Educational Activities
1. Review of Patient Transportation Safety Issues

SURGICAL SERVICES

POLICY/PROCEDURE/PROTOCOL:
Competency Assessment Plan for Pre-Operative Ambulatory Surgery

DISTRIBUTION:
Unit-Specific

PURPOSE:
To assure that all nursing staff members in the Pre-Operative Ambulatory Surgery Unit meet the identified competencies established for their job description.

POLICY:
The following competencies/educational activities will be assessed annually for each staff member:

REGISTERED NURSE
Competency Assessments
1. Interpret Selected PAT Results for Normality/Abnormality (written test)
2. Perform Peripheral Venipuncture
3. Administer IV Drugs
4. Glucose Monitoring
5. Nursing Assessment (every 2 years)
6. Peripheral IV Insertion
7. Delegating Work Assignments

NURSING TECHNICIAN
Competency Assessments
1. Taking Vital Signs
2. Obtain EKG
3. Glucose Monitoring
4. Prime and Set-Up IV Lines

NURSING ASSISTANT
Competency Assessments
1. Taking Vital Signs
2. Patient Transport
3. Waste Removal

SURGICAL SERVICES

POLICY/PROCEDURE/PROTOCOL:
Competency Assessment Plan for Post-Anesthesia Care Unit (PACU)

DISTRIBUTION:
Unit-Specific

PURPOSE:
To assure that all nursing staff members in the Post-Anesthesia Care Unit meet the identified competencies established for their job description.

POLICY:
The following competencies/educational activities will be assessed annually for each staff member:

REGISTERED NURSE
Competency Assessments
1. ABG Collection
2. Defibrillation
3. Interpretation of Life-Threatening Arrhythmias (written test)
4. Glucose Monitoring
5. Nursing Assessment (every 2 years)
6. Delegating Work Assignments

Educational Activities
1. Review of Anesthesia Drugs/Reversal Drugs
2. Review of Malignant Hyperthermia Symptomology and Treatment

NURSING TECHNICIAN
Competency Assessments
1. Obtain EKG
2. Discontinuation of IV
3. Telemetry Lead Placement
4. Taking Vital Signs
5. Glucose Monitoring
6. Patient Transport

SURGICAL SERVICES

POLICY/PROCEDURE/PROTOCOL:
Competency Assessment Plan for Post-Operative Ambulatory Surgery

DISTRIBUTION:
Unit-Specific

PURPOSE:
To assure that all nursing staff members in the Post-Operative Ambulatory Surgery Unit meet the identified competencies established for their job description.

POLICY:
The following competencies/educational activities will be assessed annually for each staff member:

REGISTERED NURSE
Competency Assessments
1. Management of Patient Requiring Post-Op Pain Medication
2. Management of Patient with Cardiac Cath with Brachial Cutdown
3. Care of the Patient Having Blood Patch Therapy
4. Glucose Monitoring
5. Nursing Assessment (every 2 years)
6. Care of the Patient Having Angiography
Educational Activities
1. Review of Anesthesia Drugs/Reversal Drugs
2. Review of Selected Cardiac Arrthymia Patterns

NURSING TECHNICIAN
Competency Assessments
1. Obtain EKG
2. Discontinuation of IV
3. Taking Vital Signs
4. Glucose Monitoring
Educational Activities
1. Review Assisting with Post-Op Ambulation

CHAPTER 4

COMPETENCY WORKSHEETS

Chapter 4

Competency Worksheets

Chapter 4 presents 190 actual competency worksheets, most of which have been piloted at least once. Please refer to the INDEX for page numbers of specific competencies.

It is imperative that staff validate the performance chosen for each competency in a particular institution. The intention is to validate staff performance, not to confuse or outwit the staff member.

NAME _____

UNIT _____

DATE _____

COMPETENCY: ABG COLLECTION—ADULT		
PERFORMANCE CRITERIA	**COMPLETED BY STAFF**	
1. Instructs patient concerning procedure.	Y	N
2. Gathers appropriate equipment.	Y	N
3. Chooses appropriate site.	Y	N
4. If using RADIAL site only, performs Allens test and states purposes.	Y	N
5. Positions selected site appropriately: RADIAL: hand supine on flat surface, slightly elevated with wrist hyperextended. BRACHIAL: arm abducted, supine and supported on flat surface. FEMORAL: leg abducted with foot everted in supine position.	Y	N
6. Prepares pre-heparinized syringe.	Y	N
7. Prepares site using sterile technique and universal precautions	Y	N
8. Palpates selected artery.	Y	N
9. Performs percutaneous puncture of selected artery with bevel up at 45 degree angle for Radial; 90 degree angle for Brachial and Femoral.	Y	N
10. Observes syringe for flashback of blood and obtains 1 to 1½ cc. of arterial blood.	Y	N
11. Applies firm pressure over puncture site with dry, sterile dressing for 5 minutes (radial/brachial sites) or 10 minutes (femoral).	Y	N
12. Expresses air from syringe sample, seals sample with a cap and immerses sample in ice.	Y	N
13. Labels sample appropriately and sends to lab STAT.	Y	N
14. Assesses site for hemorrhage. Applies pressure dressing if needed.	Y	N
COMMENTS:		

Evaluator_____

NAME _____

UNIT _____

DATE _____

COMPETENCY: Arterial Blood Gas Sampling by Respiratory Care Practitioners	
PERFORMANCE CRITERIA	COMPLETED BY STAFF
1. Checks chart to verify order.	Y N
2. Determines positive patient identification.	Y N
3. Gathers equipment utilizing Universal Precautions.	Y N
4. Explains procedure to patient.	Y N
5. Ascertains Anticoagulant Therapy.	Y N
6. Chooses appropriate site.	Y N
7. Performs Allens Test if radial site is used.	Y N
8. Prepares site using sterile technique.	Y N
9. Palpates selected artery.	Y N
10. Punctures site (45 degree for radial, 90 degree for brachial, femoral).	Y N
11. Obtains 1-1½ cc.	Y N
12. Applies pressure 5 minutes (radial/brachial sites); 10 minutes (femoral site).	Y N
13. Assesses for hemorrhage (applies pressure dressing if needed).	Y N
14. Expels air from sample; seals sample; immerses sample in ice.	Y N
15. Labels sample; obtains lab slip (includes draw site FiO_2).	Y N
16. Notifies appropriate staff to send sample to STAT Lab.	Y N
17. Documents procedure appropriately.	Y N
COMMENTS:	

Evaluator_____

NAME   _____

UNIT   _____

DATE   _____

COMPETENCY: Calculation of Absolute Neutrophile Count		
PERFORMANCE CRITERIA	**COMPLETED BY STAFF**	
1. Identifies WBC results.	Y	N
2. Identifies segs and bands levels.	Y	N
3. Uses following formula to calculate ANC: ANC = (Segs + bands) x WBC	Y	N
4. Determines if patient is at risk for infection.	Y	N
COMMENTS:		

Evaluator_____

NAME _____

UNIT _____

DATE _____

COMPETENCY: Accessing Implanted Ports		
PERFORMANCE CRITERIA	**COMPLETED BY STAFF**	
1. Washes hands. Uses well lighted area for procedure.	Y	N
2. Assembles appropriate equipment.	Y	N
3. Maintaines sterile technique throughout procedure.	Y	N
4. Primes needle extension set with saline. Prepares flush syringes with appropriate fluid.	Y	N
5. Positions patient to expose port.	Y	N
6. Palpates site to locate septum.	Y	N
7. Prepares site and access port according to protocol.	Y	N
8. Stabilizes port with one hand and inserts needle/syringe perpendicularly until it reaches the bottom of the port chamber.	Y	N
9. Checks for blood return.	Y	N
10. Flushes port and chamber with saline. Flushes port and chamber with Heparin.	Y	N
11. Assesses site for swelling or abnormal discharge.	Y	N
12. Applies sterile, transparent dressing and labels dressing appropriately.	Y	N
13. Attaches ordered fluid or adapter.	Y	N
14. Instructs patient according to unit standards.	Y	N
COMMENTS:		

Evaluator_____

82

NAME _____

UNIT _____

DATE _____

COMPETENCY: Care of the Patient having an Angiography		
PERFORMANCE CRITERIA	**COMPLETED BY STAFF**	
1. Assesses groin site for hematoma on admission.	Y	N

2. Assesses the following throughout the procedure:
  a. groin site
  b. dorsalis pedal pulse
  c. vital signs
	Y	N

3. Notifies physician of:
  a. changes in vital signs
  b. changes in dorsalis pedal pulse
  c. complaints of chest pain
  d. indications of site bleeding or increase in size of existing hematoma.
	Y	N

4. Documents all assessment data accurately on the appropriate form.	Y	N
5. Encourages fluid intake, monitoring patient's tolerance to fluids and solids intake.	Y	N
6. Maintains IV access throughout procedure.	Y	N
7. Assists patient OOB, assessing tolerance to ambulation, after physician exam.	Y	N
8. Assesses groin site, vital signs prior to discharge.	Y	N

9. Provides patient discharge instructions:
  a. written instructions for care of groin site
  b. appropriate actions to take if bleeding occurs
	Y	N

COMMENTS:		

Evaluator_____

NAME _____

UNIT _____

DATE _____

COMPETENCY: Angiography/Cardiac Catherization Circulating		
PERFORMANCE CRITERIA	**COMPLETED BY STAFF**	
1. Places patient's medical record number on film.	Y	N
2. Educates patient regarding exam.	Y	N
3. Documents patient education.	Y	N
4. Sets proper technique (line, overhead).	Y	N
5. Sets proper injection flow rate.	Y	N
6. Sets proper film rate.	Y	N
7. Cleans exam table according to department standard and provides clean linen for each patient.	Y	N
8. Documents all pertinent information regarding procedure.	Y	N
9. Turns room around in timely manner.	Y	N
COMMENTS:		

Evaluator_____

NAME _____
UNIT _____
DATE _____

COMPETENCY: Angiography/Cardiac Catheterization Scrubbing Technique		
PERFORMANCE CRITERIA	**COMPLETED BY STAFF**	
1. Performs surgical scrub according to policy.	Y	N
2. Maintains sterile technique throughout procedure.	Y	N
3. Sets up table according to department standards.	Y	N
4. Identifies all instruments and supplies necessary for all exams.	Y	N
5. Places gown and sterile gloves on, using sterile technique.	Y	N
6. Cleans table and instruments according to department standards.	Y	N
COMMENTS:		

Evaluator_____

NAME _____

UNIT _____

DATE _____

COMPETENCY: Assessment and Immediate Treatment of Extravasation of Chemotherapeutic Agents		
PERFORMANCE CRITERIA	COMPLETED BY STAFF	
1. Visually inspects site for: a. redness at the site b. swelling at the site or of the extremity c. leakage of fluid or bleeding at the site	Y	N
2. Palpates for induration, edema and changes in temperature.	Y	N
3. Checks for tenderness/pain and blood return in IV tubing.	Y	N
4. If extravasation is suspected: a. Discontinues chemotherapy leaving needle/catheter in place. b. Aspirates residual medication and blood. c. Applies ice to IV site except when chemo agent is vinca alkyloid. d. Notifies physician immediately.	Y	N
5. If extravastion is diagnosed: a. Applies treatment as ordered. b. Discontinues IV if treatment does not need it. c. Elevates extremity.	Y	N
6. Restarts IV in other extremity or proximal to extravasation site.	Y	N
7. Documents according to Structure Standards.	Y	N
COMMENTS:		

Evaluator_____

NAME   _____

UNIT   _____

DATE   _____

COMPETENCY: Cardiovascular Assessment (General)		
PERFORMANCE CRITERIA	**COMPLETED BY STAFF**	
1. Participant assesses patient history for cardiac problems and medications.	Y	N
2. Participant correctly identifies selected anatomical landmarks.	Y	N
3. Participant uses correct technique to assess the Central Cardiac System including:	Y	N
Heart Rate and Rhythm	Y	N
Heart Sounds	Y	N
Capillary Refill	Y	N
Apical and Peripheral Pulses	Y	N
Edema	Y	N
Skin Temperature	Y	N
Skin Color	Y	N
4. Participant utilizes correct techniques to assess the peripheral vascular system.	Y	N
5. Participant correctly differentiates between normal and ABN findings.	Y	N
6. Participant correctly differentiates between normal and ABN ECG patterns.	Y	N
7. Participant correctly identifies lab results which have a negative impact on the Cardiovascular System.	Y	N
8. Participant identifies appropriate nursing dignoses from findings.	Y	N
9. Participant appropriately documents findings.	Y	N
COMMENTS:		

Evaluator_____

NAME   _____

UNIT   _____

DATE   _____

COMPETENCY: Complete Nursing Assessment		
PERFORMANCE CRITERIA	**COMPLETED BY STAFF**	
1. Participant assesses for Psychosocial needs.	Y	N
2. Participant assesses for educational needs of:		
Patient	Y	N
Family	Y	N
3. Participant assesses for spiritual needs of:		
Patient	Y	N
Family	Y	N
4. Participant follows up on ABN history findings.	Y	N
5. Participant completes a head-to-toe assessment using correct techiques for:		
Inspection	Y	N
Palpation	Y	N
Persussion	Y	N
Auscultation	Y	N
6. Participant examines diagnostic studies for ABN findings which negatively impact health.	Y	N
7. Participant refer ABN findings of the Nursing Assessment to the appropriate health care team member.	Y	N
COMMENTS:		

Evaluator_____

Copy for Don

NAME _____ ____
UNIT _____
DATE _____

COMPETENCY: Education Assessment of Patients and Families		
PERFORMANCE CRITERIA	COMPLETED BY STAFF	
1. Assesses willingness to learn.	Y	N
2. Assesses ability to learn.	Y	N
3. Assesses for barriers to learning including:	Y	N
a. anxiety	Y	N
b. pain	Y	N
c. fatigue	Y	N
d. memory loss	Y	N
e. denial	Y	N
f. anger	Y	N
4. Assesses knowledge base of specific educational components including:	Y	N
a. current health problesm	Y	N
b. self care	Y	N
c. safe use of medications	Y	N
d. therapuetic nutrition and diet	Y	N
e. follow-up care	Y	N
f. on-going health care needs	Y	N
g. choices of options/consequences of choices	Y	N
5. Identifies misinformation	Y	N
6. Includes members of the support system when appropriate.	Y	N
7. Documents findings in the medical record.	Y	N
COMMENTS:		

Evaluator_____

NAME   _____

UNIT   _____

DATE   _____

COMPETENCY: Gastrointestinal Assessment		
PERFORMANCE CRITERIA	**COMPLETED BY STAFF**	
1. Participant identifies selected anatomical landmarks.	Y	N
2. Participant assesses history for complaints of GI origin.	Y	N
3. Participant utilizes correct technique to assess:		
Oral Cavity	Y	N
ABD Symmetry/Contour/Shape	Y	N
Masses/Pulsation	Y	N
Bowel Sounds	Y	N
4. Participant correctly differentiates between normal and ABN bowel sounds.	Y	N
5. Participant correctly differentiates between normal and ABN percussion results.	Y	N
6. Participant correctly uses technique of light palpation.	Y	N
7. Participant uses correct technique for deep palpation.	Y	N
8. Participant correctly identifies ABN exam findings.	Y	N
9. Participant identifies ABN diagnostic studies which effect the GI System.	Y	N
10. Participant identifies appropriate nursing diagnoses from data.	Y	N
11. Participant appropriately documents findings.		
COMMENTS:		

Evaluator_____

NAME   _____

UNIT   _____

DATE   _____

COMPETENCY: Genito-urinary Assessment		
PERFORMANCE CRITERIA	**COMPLETED BY STAFF**	
1. Participant correctly identifies selected anatomical landmarks.	Y	N
2. Participant assesses for past history impacting the GU System.	Y	N
3. Participant uses correct techniques to assess:		
Masses/Edema	Y	N
Positon of Urethral Opening	Y	N
Incisional Lines	Y	N
Exudates	Y	N
Bladder Distention	Y	N
Genitalia	Y	N
Herniations	Y	N
4. Participant identifies ABN diagnostic rsults which impact the GU System.	Y	N
5. Participant identifies appropriate nursing diagnosis from findings.	Y	N
6. Participant correctly documents findings.	Y	N
COMMENTS:		

Evaluator_____

NAME _____

UNIT _____

DATE _____

COMPETENCY: Inital Post-delivery Newborn Assessment		
PERFORMANCE CRITERIA	**COMPLETED BY STAFF**	
1. Scores newborn accurately using Apgar criteria at 1 minute.	Y	N
2. Scores newborn accurately using Apgar criteria at 5 minutes.	Y	N
3. Recognizes abnormal cardiac activity.	Y	N
4. Assesses for signs and symptoms of respiratory distress.	Y	N
5. Uses bulb syringe properly.	Y	N
6. Suctions via catheter appropriately.	Y	N
7. Clamps cord according to policy.	Y	N
8. Assesses both fontanelles for size and pulse.	Y	N
9. Recognizes normal variations in skin color.	Y	N
10. Implements chemstick protocols when appropriate.	Y	N
11. Demonstrates proper technique for IM injections of Vitamin K.	Y	N
12. Demonstrates proper technique in placing Erythromycin Ointment in eyes of neonate.	Y	N
13. Obtains accurate birth weight using electronic scale.	Y	N
14. Determines the SGA-AGA-LGA status of infant.	Y	N
15. Identifies signs/symptoms of hypo- or hyperglycemic states in neonate.	Y	N
16. Implements thermostability.	Y	N
17. Identifies positive/negative bonding behaviors between infant and mother.	Y	N
18. Assesses for neurological reflexes which confirm absence of neuro injury/disease.	Y	N
19. Reports significant findings to nursing staff at time of transfer.	Y	N
COMMENTS:		

Evaluator_____

NAME   _____

UNIT   _____

DATE   _____

COMPETENCY: IV Site Assessment		
PERFORMANCE CRITERIA	**COMPLETED BY STAFF**	
1. If dressing is NOT transparent, remove it and discard appropriately without removing the tape securing the IV.	Y	N

2.   Visually inspect the site for:
   a. redness at the site or a red streak up the arm
   b. swelling of the site or extremity
   c. pallor at the site
   d. leakage of fluid or drainage
	Y	N

3. Palpate for induration, edema and changes in temperature.	Y	N
4. Check for tenderness/pain and blood return.	Y	N
5. Document all findings.	Y	N
COMMENTS:		

Evaluator_____

NAME _____

UNIT _____

DATE _____

COMPETENCY: Musculoskeletal Assessment		
PERFORMANCE CRITERIA	**COMPLETED BY STAFF**	
1. Participant identifies function of selected anatomical structures/landmarkes.	Y	N
2. Participant assesses head and neck for:		
Symmetry	Y	N
Size	Y	N
Contour	Y	N
ROM	Y	N
Involuntary Movements	Y	N
3. Participant assesses spine for:		
Contour	Y	N
Position	Y	N
Motion	Y	N
Tenderness	Y	N
4. Participant uses correct technique in assessing motor function and strength of:		
Upper Extremities	Y	N
Lower Extremities	Y	N
5. Participant refers ABN findingsto the appropriate healthcare team member.	Y	N
6. Participant appropriately documents findings.	Y	N
7. Participant identifies appropriate nursing diagnoses.	Y	N
COMMENTS:		

Evaluator_____

NAME _____

UNIT _____

DATE _____

COMPETENCY: Newborn Assessment		
PERFORMANCE CRITERIA	**COMPLETED BY STAFF**	
1. Identifies thermostability in neonate.	Y	N
2. Identifies respiratory rate and presence/absence of respiratory distress.	Y	N
3. Recognizes normal/abnormal cardiac activity.	Y	N
4. Recognizes normal variations in neonate skin color and integrity.	Y	N
5. Identifies signs/symptoms of hypo- and hyperglycemic states.	Y	N
6. Implements chem protocols when appropriate.	Y	N

7. Identifies infant's abilities on the following:
  a. voiding patterns
  b. stool patterns
  c. feeding patterns, determining whether it is within the acceptable range.
	Y	N

8. Recognizes signs/symptoms of over- and under-feeding.	Y	N
9. Assessses the appearance of infant's potential infectious sites, including circumcision and umbilical cord.	Y	N
10. Identifies positive/negative Mother/Infant bonding.	Y	N
11. Identifies the infant's behavioral state.	Y	N
12. Identifies signs/symptoms of probable withdrawal.	Y	N
13. Identifies actual and potential problems based on the assessment.	Y	N
145. Documents assessment appropriately.		
COMMENTS:		

Evaluator_____

NAME _____

UNIT _____

DATE _____

COMPETENCY: Neurological Assessment		
PERFORMANCE CRITERIA	**COMPLETED BY STAFF**	
1. Participant assesses for past history of neurological problems.	Y	N
2. Participant utilizes correct techniques to assess:		
Mental Status	Y	N
Speech and Language Function	Y	N
Cranial Nerve Function	Y	N
Proprioception	Y	N
Cerebellar Function	Y	N
Sensory Function	Y	N
Reflexes	Y	N
3. Participant carries out a complete NSDO (neuro check).	Y	N
4. Participant differentiates between normal and ABN findings.	Y	N
5. Participant identifies appropriate nursing diagnoses from findings.	Y	N
6. Participants appropriately documents findings.	Y	N
COMMENTS:		

Evaluator_____

NAME _____

UNIT _____

DATE _____

COMPETENCY: Nursing Assessment--Endoscopy		
PERFORMANCE CRITERIA	COMPLETED BY STAFF	
1. Completes endoscopy preoperative nursing assessment document prior to procedure.	Y	N
2. Documents baseline ABD assessment prior to endoscopy.	Y	N
3. Correctly applies cardiac monitor prior to procedure and obtains baseline ECG tracing.	Y	N
4. Monitors cardiac status throughout procedure.	Y	N
5. Assesses skin color and temperature periodically throughout procedure and post-operatively.	Y	N
6. Monitors vital signs every 3 minutes and records them every 15 minutes.	Y	N
COMMENTS:		

Evaluator_____

NAME   _____

UNIT   _____

DATE   _____

COMPETENCY: Nursing Assessment of the Ambulatory OB Patient		
PERFORMANCE CRITERIA	COMPLETED BY STAFF	
1. Validates patient's responses on prenatal nursing assessment questionnaire.	Y	N
2. Verifies written documentation of positive pregnancy status by serum HCG, sonogram, or fetal heart tones.	Y	N
3. Identifies approximate gestional age and EDC based on LMP.	Y	N
4. Assesses reproductive history including parity.	Y	N
5. Assesses support system.	Y	N
6. Assesses patient response/desire to continue pregnancy.	Y	N
7. Assesses patient's SES and educational status.	Y	N

8.   Identifies SES and educational related needs including:
    a.   Nutrition
    b.   Transportation
    c.   Schools
    d.   Activity
    e.   Health needs
    f.   Employment
    g.   Pregnancy or prenatal care related issues according to structure standards.
	Y	N

9. Assesses risk for pregnancy complication or exacerbation of existing medical/psychiatric conditions.	Y	N
10. Identifies need for referrals.	Y	N
11. Assesses patient for substance abuse.	Y	N
12. Documents assessment according to unit standards.	Y	N
COMMENTS:		

Evaluator_____

NAME _____

UNIT _____

DATE _____

COMPETENCY: Assessment of Suicidal Risk		
PERFORMANCE CRITERIA	**COMPLETED BY STAFF**	
1. Monitors the patient for passive and active sucidal ideations Q shift.	Y	N
2. Monitors non-verbal behavior for suicidal risk Q shift.	Y	N
3. Assesses mood/affect especially following family or group therapy.	Y	N
4. Monitors changes in behavior Q shift.	Y	N
5. Monitors changes in energy levels.	Y	N
6. Does mouth checks after medicaton administration.	Y	N
7. Checks lab results of blood levels of prescribed medications as ordered.	Y	N
8. Documents suicide assessment Q shift.	Y	N
COMMENTS:		

Evaluator_____

NAME   _____
UNIT   _____
DATE   _____

COMPETENCY: Physical Assessment of Danger Signs for Eating Disorders	
PERFORMANCE CRITERIA	**COMPLETED BY STAFF**
1. Assesses the patient Q shift for the following 　　a. Abdominal pain 　　b. Bowel movements 　　c. Voiding 　　d. Chest pain/palpitations 　　e. 2+ pitting edema of feet and legs 　　f. Dystonic reactions 　　g. Changes in mental status 　　h. Orthostatic pulses 　　i. Skin rash	Y　　N
2. Identifies lab values which indicate potential treatment risk including K+, WBC, SGOT/SGPT, serum glucose and HCG.	Y　　N
3. Documents finding according to unit policy.	Y　　N
COMMENTS:	

Evaluator_____

NAME _____

UNIT _____

DATE _____

COMPETENCY: Postpartum Maternal Assessment		
PERFORMANCE CRITERIA	**COMPLETED BY STAFF**	
1. Explains procedure to patient.	Y	N
2. Maintains adequate privacy throughout procedure.	Y	N
3. Verbally assesses for pain or discomfort.	Y	N
4. Identifies the following:		
a. Breast changes	Y	N
b. Involutional status including fundal and lochial status	Y	N
c. Voiding behaviors and bladder status	Y	N
d. Vital signs	Y	N
e. Educational needs for this family	Y	N
f. Stage of psychological adjustment to maternal role	Y	N
5. Assesses the following:		
a. Bowel function appropriate for type of delivery	Y	N
b. Pulmonary function on Ceasarean section patients	Y	N
c. Recovery from anesthesia	Y	N
d. Episiotomy and/or incisional site using REEDA scale		
e. Thrombophlebotic status		
f. Fluid shift stage		
6. Compares all data to the expections for that postpartal stage.		
COMMENTS:		

Evaluator_____

NAME _____

UNIT _____

DATE _____

COMPETENCY: Psychosocial Assessment of Clients		
PERFORMANCE CRITERIA	**COMPLETED BY STAFF**	
1. Introduces self to client.	Y	N
2. Explains purpose of assessment to client.	Y	N
3. Identifies client's normal coping pattern.	Y	N
4. Identifies major stressors in client's life.	Y	N
5. Assesses communication style.	Y	N
6. Assesses mental status including:		
a. mood and affect	Y	N
b. orientation to person, place, time and circumstances	Y	N
c. attention span	Y	N
d. Perceptual distortions	Y	N
e. thought processes	Y	N
7. Assesses social network including:		
a. local support persons	Y	N
b. emergency contacts	Y	N
c. other visitors	Y	N
8. Assesses socio-economic status including:		
a. employment	Y	N
b. cultural and ethnic identification	Y	N
c. strength of religious beliefs	Y	N
d. economic needs	Y	N
9. Assesses lifestyle including:		
a. family and work roles	Y	N
b. health habits	Y	N
c. residence	Y	N
d. cultural beliefs	Y	N
COMMENTS:		

Evaluator_____

NAME   _____

UNIT   _____

DATE   _____

COMPETENCY: Respiratory Assessment		
PERFORMANCE CRITERIA	**COMPLETED BY STAFF**	
1. Participant correctly identifies selected anatomical landmarks.	Y	N
2. Participant assesses for history of:		
Pulmonary Disease	Y	N
Surgeries	Y	N
Smoking	Y	N
Environmental Hazards for Respiration	Y	N
Cough	Y	N
SOB	Y	N
Pain During Respiration	Y	N
3. Participant uses correct technique to assess:		
Rate of Respiration	Y	N
Rhythm of Respiration	Y	N
Quality of Respiration	Y	N
Skin Color	Y	N
Breath Sounds	Y	N
4. Participant correctly differentiates between normal and adventitious sounds.	Y	N
5. Participant identifies appropriate nursing diagnoses from data.	Y	N
6. Participant appropriately documents data.	Y	N
COMMENTS:		

Evaluator_____

NAME _____

UNIT _____

DATE _____

COMPETENCY: Physical Assessment of the Skin	
PERFORMANCE CRITERIA	**COMPLETED BY STAFF**
1. Participant assesses current and past history of skin problems.	Y N
2. Participant assesses self treatment of skin problems (including medications).	Y N
3. Participant assesses psychosocial factors which impact skin (habits, family history, travel, occupation).	Y N
4. Participant inspects skin for:	
Color	Y N
Texture	Y N
Odor	Y N
Signs of aging	Y N
Lesions/ Rashes	Y N
Abnormal Conditions	Y N
5. Participant correctly identifies the phase of healing of any wounds.	Y N
6. Participant inspects for abnormalities of:	
Hair/Scalp	Y N
Nails	Y N
7. Participant appropriately documents data.	
COMMENTS:	

Evaluator_____

NAME _____
UNIT _____
DATE _____

COMPETENCY: Spiritual Assessment of Clients	
PERFORMANCE CRITERIA	**COMPLETED BY STAFF**
1. Identifies patient's concept of Diety or source of strength and hope.	Y N
2. Assesses patient's perception of their purpose in life.	Y N
3. Assesses meaning of hospitalization to patient and family.	Y N
4. Assesses patient's perception of the relationship between spiritual beliefs and health status.	Y N
5. Assesses significance of religious practices to patient and family.	Y N
6. Identifies need for referral to clergy when appropriate.	Y N
COMMENTS:	

Evaluator_____

NAME _____

UNIT _____

DATE _____

COMPETENCY: Assisting Physician With Medical Procedure		
PERFORMANCE CRITERIA	**COMPLETED BY STAFF**	
1. Assembles appropriate equipment.	Y	N
2. Prepares informed consent form for signatures.	Y	N
3. Maintains patient position appropriately for procedure.	Y	N
4. Maintains patient privacy throughout procedure, including proper draping.	Y	N
5. Passes equipment according to unit standards.	Y	N
6. Disposes of equipment according to unit standards.	Y	N
7. Assists patients to dress.	Y	N
8. Verifies that patient has a follow-up appointment with a physician.	Y	N
COMMENTS:		

Evaluator_____

NAME _____

UNIT _____

DATE _____

COMPETENCY: Utilization of Athrombic Pump/Anti-embolism Stockings		
PERFORMANCE CRITERIA	**COMPLETED BY STAFF**	
1. Validates physician order for anti-embolism device.	Y	N
2. Applies correctly sized anti-embolism stockings to patient: a. Measures appropriate circumference and length of patient's leg b. Orders appropriate stockings c. Correctly applies stockings to patient with feet elevated d. Removes wrinkles from stockings e. Documents date and time stockings were applied	Y	N
3. Applies arthrombic pump correctly: a. Positions inflation deices and tightens straps appropriately b. Correctly assembles tubing c. Correctly positions pump to avoid obstruction or damage to pump d. Turns pump on and assesses proper functioning	Y	N
4. Assesses circulation to extremities according to structure standards.	Y	N
COMMENTS:		

Evaluator_____

NAME _____

UNIT _____

DATE _____

COMPETENCY: Audiometric Screening		
PERFORMANCE CRITERIA	**COMPLETED BY STAFF**	
1. Controls noise level.	Y	N
2. Seats patients so that they cannot watch hand movement of tester during testing.	Y	N
3. Explains procedure to patients, instructing them to signal which ear they hear the tone.	Y	N
4. Places head phones on ears appropriately: red phone in right ear and blue phone in left ear.	Y	N
5. Dials settings: a. Tone = on b. Output = dial according to ear testing c. Masking = off d. Monitor = on	Y	N
6. Holds bar in center of audiometer to prevent patient from hearing tone; releases bar when ready to test ear.	Y	N
7. Tests both ears to 1000, 2000 & 4000 Herz. Tests 1000 and 2000 HZ starting at 20 db until patients indicate they can hear tone, raising db at increments of 5. Tests 4000 HZ beginning at 25 db until patients indicate they can hear tone, raising db at increments of 5.	Y	N
8. Records all findings as indicated on patient's chart, including db heard, if above standard.	Y	N
9. Notifies physician of any abnormalities or concerns.	Y	N
COMMENTS:		

Evaluator_____

108

NAME _____

UNIT _____

DATE _____

COMPETENCY: Use of Audio Visual Equipment		
PERFORMANCE CRITERIA	**COMPLETED BY STAFF**	
1. Gathers needed A-V equipment.	Y	N
2. Tests for proper operation of equipment.	Y	N
3. Delivers equipment to appropriate personnel/place.	Y	N
4. Instructs user on the operationof equipment.	Y	N
5. Troubleshoots minor problems with equipment.	Y	N
6. Arrange for equipment to be repaid if needed.	Y	N
COMMENTS:		

Evaluator_____

NAME _____

UNIT _____

DATE _____

COMPETENCY: Autovac Preparation	
PERFORMANCE CRITERIA	**COMPLETED BY STAFF**
1. Maintains sterile technique during transfer of tubing and canister for circulator.	Y N
2. Removes trocar cover safely.	Y N
3. Safely passes trocar with drainage tubing to surgeon.	Y N
4. Retrieves trocar safely.	Y N
5. Places trocar in needle counter.	Y N
6. Injects anticoagulant into autovac canister, using the appropriate port as ordered.	Y N
7. Marks designated area on canister with date, time of institution and amount of additive.	Y N
8. Disposes trocar, according to unit standards.	Y N
COMMENTS:	

Evaluator_____

NAME   _____

UNIT   _____

DATE   _____

COMPETENCY: Performs Modified Barium Swallow Study		
PERFORMANCE CRITERIA	**COMPLETED BY STAFF**	
1. Places patient in appropriate position.	Y	N

2. Tests consistency of:
    a. thin barium
    b. thick barium
    c. puree with barium
    d. chewable if applicable
	Y	N

3. Documents results of swallow study.	Y	N
4. Makes diet recommendations.	Y	N
5. Informs physician of results immediately following the test.	Y	N
COMMENTS:		

Evaluator_____

NAME _____

UNIT _____

DATE _____

COMPETENCY: CT Biopsy/Drainage Procedures		
PERFORMANCE CRITERIA	**COMPLETED BY STAFF**	
1. Checks patient's PT & PTT day prior to exam.	Y	N
2. Sets up table according to department standard using sterile technique.	Y	N
3. Consults with radiologist prior to exam for necessary equipment needed or special instructions.	Y	N
4. Explains procedure to patient and documents patient education.	Y	N
5. Documents history assessment.	Y	N
6. Notifies Pathology Department and Recovery Room prior to exam.	Y	N
7. Follows post exam procedures per department protocol.	Y	N
8. Documents all pertinent information.	Y	N
COMMENTS:		

Evaluator_____

NAME   _____
UNIT   _____
DATE   _____

COMPETENCY: Continuous Bladder Irrigation		
PERFORMANCE CRITERIA	**COMPLETED BY STAFF**	
1. Obtains physician's order for CBI drip rate.	Y	N
2. Ensures catheter stabilization during patient movement.	Y	N
3. Assesses I & O, color, odor and appearance of drainage during the following: a. on admission b. 30 minutes after admission c. 60 minutes after admission d. every 1 hr x 4 hours e. every 4 hours thereafter	Y	N
4. Maintains flow rate to keep I & O equal.	Y	N
5. If intake and output are equal but output is dark in color, increases flow rate p.r.n. so that output is clear, pink in color. Maintains flow rate to keep output clear.	Y	N
6. Assesses need for manual irrigation.	Y	N
7. Provides peri-care and catheter care p.r.n.	Y	N
8. Empties drainage bag each time new fluid bottle is hung.	Y	N
9. Maintains drainage bag below bladder level throughout the procedure.	Y	N
COMMENTS:		

Evaluator_____

NAME _____

UNIT _____

DATE _____

COMPETENCY: Assisting With Chest Tube Insertion (NICU)		
PERFORMANCE CRITERIA	**COMPLETED BY STAFF**	
1. Assesses patient for possible pneumo- or hemothorax.	Y	N
2. Asse,bles equipment for insertion AND drainage system, including Emerson adapter, maintaining sterile technique.	Y	N
3. Restrains infant and attaches infant to cardiac/apnea monitor.	Y	N
4. Assists physician with insertion of chest tube, maintaining sterile technique.	Y	N
5. Attaches chest drainage system to chest tube connector and suction device.	Y	N
6. Sets negative suction regulator to amount ordered.	Y	N
7. Secures all tubing and connections with tape.	Y	N
8. Documents per unit standards.	Y	N
COMMENTS:		

Evaluator_____

114

NAME _____

UNIT _____

DATE _____

COMPETENCY: Immediate Post Operative Care of Patient with Blood Patch Therapy		
PERFORMANCE CRITERIA	**COMPLETED BY STAFF**	
1. Applies Dynamap and takes baseline vital signs including temperature.	Y	N
2. Maintains patient in 30 degree upright position.	Y	N
3. Assesses patient response to blood patch: a. Changes in headache b. presence of nausea or vomiting	Y	N
4. Provides patient with fluids and encourages at least 300 cc p.o.	Y	N
5. Takes vital signs as ordered.	Y	N
6. Assists patient OOB; assesses gait and intensity of headache.	Y	N
7. Provides written copy of discharge instruction.	Y	N
COMMENTS:		

Evaluator_____

NAME _____

UNIT _____

DATE _____

COMPETENCY: PKU Blood Draw		
PERFORMANCE CRITERIA	**COMPLETED BY STAFF**	
1. Validates presence of parental consent form.	Y	N
2. Notifies pediatrician of parental refusal.	Y	N
3. Verifies accuracy of information filled in on PKU slip.	Y	N
4. Verifies correct patient.	Y	N
5. Utilizes appropriate sterile technique throughout procedure to control for infection.	Y	N
6. Selects appropriate site and prepares infant's heel for specimen collection.	Y	N
7. Completely fills all 5 circles from one side.	Y	N
8. Provides parents with reinforcement teaching regarding purpose of test.	Y	N
COMMENTS:		

Evaluator_____

NAME   _____

UNIT   _____

DATE   _____

COMPETENCY: Testing Stool of Occult Blood		
PERFORMANCE CRITERIA	**COMPLETED BY STAFF**	
1. Washes hands and puts non-sterile gloves on.	Y	N
2. Checks slide and reagent for expiration dates.	Y	N
3. Applies sufficient amount of stool to cover area on hemoccult slide.	Y	N
4. Applies reagent correctly.	Y	N
5. Reads slide within 3 seconds of required time.	Y	N
6. Accurately reads test results.	Y	N
7. Documents results and notifies RN of abnormal results.	Y	N
COMMENTS:		

Evaluator_____

NAME _____

UNIT _____

DATE _____

COMPETENCY: Transfusion of Blood and Blood Components		
PERFORMANCE CRITERIA	**COMPLETED BY STAFF**	
1. Obtains blood products from blood bank.	Y	N
2. Washes hand and dons non-sterile gloves.	Y	N
3. Obtains patient's T.P.R. and BP. [If T. is elevated to 100° or above, hold transfusion; obtains order to transfuse despite temperature]	Y	N
4. Confirms identity of patient receiving blood product by asking patient to state name and birthdate.	Y	N
5. Confirms identity of patient by checking typenex bracelet with typenex number on unit of blood.	Y	N
6. Primes the transfusion tubing with the blood or blood product. Starts and regulates the transfusion.	Y	N
7. Completes the yellow and blue transfusion records.	Y	N
8. Educates the patient regarding transfusion protocol and possible reactions.	Y	N
9. Ensures that transfusion will be complete prior to 4 hrs.	Y	N
10. Ensures that no other IV medications are infusing into the same line. [When blood is hung by unit staff, verification of blood and patient must by done by two (2) nurses]	Y	N
11. Documents appropriately.	Y	N
COMMENTS:		

Evaluator_____

NAME   _____

UNIT   _____

DATE   _____

COMPETENCY: Performs a Bone Scan		
PERFORMANCE CRITERIA	**COMPLETED BY STAFF**	
1. Washes hands and puts on non-sterile gloves.	Y	N
2. Injects the patient with the proper radiopharmaceutical.	Y	N
3. Instructs the patient properly.	Y	N
4. Places the patient on the proper scinti-bed table.	Y	N
5. Performs the bone scan according to departmental protocol.	Y	N
6. Ensures patient safety according to protocol.	Y	N
7. Develops and critique your film.	Y	N
8. Consults with the physician before you discharge the patient.	Y	N
9. Places the film and paper work in the reading room.	Y	N
COMMENTS:		

Evaluator_____

NAME _____

UNIT _____

DATE _____

COMPETENCY: Bottle Feeding Infants		
PERFORMANCE CRITERIA	**COMPLETED BY STAFF**	
1. Washes hands.	Y	N
2. Selects appropriate type and amount of formula.	Y	N
3. Holds infant firmly with head elevated.	Y	N
4. Inserts nipple into back of mouth and on top of tongue.	Y	N
5. Ensures that nipple stays full of formula while in infant's mouth.	Y	N
6. Burps infant periodically, at least halfway through and at the conclusion of feeding.	Y	N
7. Documents amount and tolerance to feeding.	Y	N
COMMENTS:		

Evaluator_____

NAME _____

UNIT _____

DATE _____

COMPETENCY: Breast Feeding Techniques		
PERFORMANCE CRITERIA	**COMPLETED BY STAFF**	
1. Identifies patient's motive for breast feeding.	Y	N
2. Identifies patient's knowledge base, discussing advantages/ disadvantages with patient.	Y	N
3. Assesses type of nipples patient has. If nipple type poses challenge to successful breastfeeding, provides teaching and support techniques.	Y	N
4. Assists mother and infant in the use of correct positioning to permit latching on. Observes mother during breastfeeding for use of feeding positions.	Y	N
5. Observes the following during nursing: a. Nasal area cleared for infant's breathing b. Positioning so traction not applied to nipple c. Correct sucking technique	Y	N
6. Identifies length of feeding time and provides mother with feedback regarding length and frequency of feeding.	Y	N
7. Explains to mother "nipple confusion" efforts upon breastfeeding.	Y	N
8. Provides mother with resource help for breastfeeding during hospital stay and after discharge.	Y	N
9. Provides information to mother regarding how to tell if the infant is receiving enough intake from breast.	Y	N
COMMENTS:		

Evaluator_____

NAME _____

UNIT _____

DATE _____

COMPETENCY: Immediate Post-Operative Care of the Cardiac Catheterization Patient with a Brachial Cut-down.		
PERFORMANCE CRITERIA	**COMPLETED BY STAFF**	
1. Applies Dynamap and gets baseline vital signs including temperature.	Y	N
2. Checks radial pulse in involved arm for presence/absence, strength and volume.	Y	N
3. Assesses dressing security and presence of drainage or hemorrhage.	Y	N
4. Notifies physician of: a. change in radial pulse volume, strength b. complaints of chest pain c. hemorrhage at cut-down site	Y	N
5. Documents vital signs (P, BP, R) every 15 minutes.	Y	N
6. Assists with OOB, assesses gait and tolerance to ambulation.	Y	N
7. Provides written copy of discharge instructions for the care of cut-down site.	Y	N
COMMENTS:		

Evaluator_____

NAME   _____

UNIT   _____

DATE   _____

COMPETENCY: Bronchial Hygiene		
PERFORMANCE CRITERIA	**COMPLETED BY STAFF**	
1. Ascertains appropriate physician order.	Y	N
2. Identifies indications for non-routine precautions.	Y	N
3. Gathers appropriate equipment for prescribed therapy.	Y	N
4. Explains procedure to patient.	Y	N
5. Positions patient optimally, as therapy indicates.	Y	N
6. Assesses patient before, during and after therapy.	Y	N
7. Observes for any adverse reactions during therapy.	Y	N
8. Documents procedure appropriately.	Y	N
COMMENTS:		

Evaluator_____

NAME _____

UNIT _____

DATE _____

COMPETENCY: Carotid Magnetic Resonance Angiography (MRA) Protocols		
PERFORMANCE CRITERIA	**COMPLETED BY STAFF**	
1. Identifies patient.	Y	N
2. Educates patient regarding exam.	Y	N
3. Documents patient's education.	Y	N
4. Chooses appropriate coil according to patient's body habitus.	Y	N
5. Chooses appropraite scanning protocol.	Y	N
6. Performs Multi Image Planer (MIP) on acquired data.	Y	N
7. Reconstructs images for hard copy films.	Y	N
8. Documents all pertinent information according to department policy.	Y	N
COMMENTS:		

Evaluator_____

NAME   _____

UNIT   _____

DATE   _____

COMPETENCY: Declotting Central Venous Catheters using Urokinase		
PERFORMANCE CRITERIA	**COMPLETED BY STAFF**	
1. Validates physician's order.	Y	N
2. Assembles appropriate equipment.	Y	N
3. Explains procedure to patient.	Y	N
4. Determines catheter occulusion by attempting to aspirate blood using a 10cc syringe.	Y	N
5. Attaches appropriate size syringe prefilled with Urokinase to catheter hub.	Y	N
6. Slowly injects ordered dose of Urokinase into catheter.	Y	N
7. Clamps Central Line, leaving syringe attached to catheter hub. After 5 minutes, check for blood return.	Y	N
8. If blood return, gently aspirate clot residual, Urokinase and 4-5ml of blood (aspiration may be attempted every 5 minutes x 30 minutes).	Y	N
9. If patency is not restored; administers 2nd dose.	Y	N
10. After patency established - remove blood filled syringe and replaces with saline filled syringe and gently flushes catheter.	Y	N
11. Replaces injection cap (if removed) and resumes ordered therapy or flushes with 3cc 1:100 heparin.	Y	N
COMMENTS:		

Evaluator_____

NAME   _____

UNIT   _____

DATE   _____

COMPETENCY: Drawing Blood From Central Lines		
PERFORMANCE CRITERIA	**COMPLETED BY STAFF**	
1. Washes hands. Uses a clean, well-lighted areas for procedure.	Y	N
2. Assembles appropriate equipment.	Y	N
3. Maintains sterile technique throughout procedure. Dons clean gloves.	Y	N
4. Stops all infusions for one minute.	Y	N
5. Clamps catheter lumen being used (not necessary for Groshongs).	Y	N
6. Removes luer-lock cap and attaches vacutainer/syringe.	Y	N
7. Draws 5 to 10 cc of discard specimen (30 cc if PT/PTT is being tested).	Y	N
8. Obtains specimen sample.	Y	N
9. Flushes port with appropriate fluid(s).	Y	N
10. Reconnects infusion or sterile luer-lock cap.	Y	N
11. Labels specimen appropriately and prepares specimen for transport maintaining universal precautions.	Y	N
COMMENTS:		

Evaluator_____

NAME _____

UNIT _____

DATE _____

COMPETENCY: Central Line Maintenance		
PERFORMANCE CRITERIA	**COMPLETED BY STAFF**	
1. Washes hands. Uses a clean, well-lighted area for procedure.	Y	N
2. Assembles appropriate equipment.	Y	N
3. Maintains sterile technique throughout procedure. Dons sterile gloves.	Y	N
4. Assesses site for complications.	Y	N
5. Prepares site according to policy, allowing site to air dry after application of liquid antispetic (e.g. Betadine).	Y	N
6. Applies antibiotic ointment p.r.n.	Y	N
7. Applies appropriate skin preparation.	Y	N
8. Applies sterile, transparent dressing over site (e.g. Tegaderm).	Y	N
9. Labels new dressing appropriately.	Y	N
10. Documents site care including observations of insertion site (e.g. presence of drainage, color, odor, etc.).	Y	N
11. Educates patient and reinforces education on central line maintenance.	Y	N
COMMENTS:		

Evaluator_____

NAME _____

UNIT _____

DATE _____

COMPETENCY: Assisting With Collection of Cervical Specimens		
PERFORMANCE CRITERIA	**COMPLETED BY STAFF**	
1. Assembles appropriate equipment for the specific procedure.	Y	N
2. Prelabels all specimen containers.	Y	N
3. Prepares speculum and conveys it to care provider.	Y	N
4. Passes collection containers to care provider.	Y	N
5. Receives specimens from care provider.	Y	N
6. Appropriately packages specimens for transport to lab.	Y	N
7. Disposes of equipment and supplies according to unit standards.	Y	N
COMMENTS:		

Evaluator_____

NAME _____
UNIT _____
DATE _____

COMPETENCY: Cervical Spine Radiograph		
PERFORMANCE CRITERIA	**COMPLETED BY STAFF**	
1. Calls patient by name.	Y	N
2. Correlates clinical indicators for exam with exam ordered.	Y	N
3. Educates patient regarding exam.	Y	N
4. Removes any clothing, dentures, earrings, necklaces, etc. if necessary.	Y	N
5. Sets proper technique.	Y	N
6. Demonstrates proper positioning skills.	Y	N
7. Logs exam in computer.	Y	N
8. Documents all pertinent information on requisitions.	Y	N
9. Follows department standards for post exam activities (i.e. logging film. patient instructions, etc.).	Y	N
COMMENTS:		

Evaluator_____

NAME _____
UNIT _____
DATE _____

COMPETENCY: Chart Assembly		
PERFORMANCE CRITERIA	**COMPLETED BY STAFF**	
1. Stamps each sheet in the chart with patient's address-o-graph card.	Y	N
2. Inserts pages into chart in correct order.	Y	N
3. Inserts dividers into chart in correct order.	Y	N
4. Labels chart on front and side binders appropriately.	Y	N
5. Disassembles chart in correct order.	Y	N
COMMENTS:		

Evaluator_____

NAME   _____

UNIT   _____

DATE   _____

COMPETENCY: Charting Intake and Output (I & O)		
PERFORMANCE CRITERIA	COMPLETED BY STAFF	
1. Verifies patient's name on I & O worksheet.	Y	N
2. Records actual amount and type of fluid intake at time of intake.	Y	N
3. Records actual amount and type of output at time of output.	Y	N
4. Records data in correct section for shift and type of data.	Y	N
5. Totals all columns at end of shift correctly.	Y	N
6. Records shift totals on TPR flowsheet.	Y	N
7. Notifies RN of shift totals prior to report.	Y	N
8. Identifies patient populations which should receive I & O monitoring: a. All medical patients b. All postoperative patients x 48 hrs c. All ICU/CCU patients d. All patients with NGT, Foley Caths, or IVs e. All patients with physician's order for I & O	Y	N
COMMENTS:		

Evaluator_____

NAME   _____

UNIT   _____

DATE   _____

COMPETENCY: Immediate Response to Chemotherapy Spill		
PERFORMANCE CRITERIA	**COMPLETED** **BY STAFF**	
1. Recognizes a spill.	Y	N
2. Obtains Chemo Spill Kit.	Y	N
3. Protects patient's skin from spill.	Y	N
4. Notifies nurse of spill.	Y	N
COMMENTS:		

Evaluator_____

NAME   _____

UNIT   _____

DATE   _____

COMPETENCY: Managing a Chemotherapy Spill		
PERFORMANCE CRITERIA	COMPLETED BY STAFF	
1. Obtains Chemo Spill Kit.	Y	N
2. Secures area.	Y	N
3. Calculates amount of spill.	Y	N
4. Notifies housekeeping of spill.	Y	N
5. Files incident report.	Y	N
6. Reassures patient.	Y	N
7. Notifies pharmacy of amount spilled.	Y	N
8. Notifies physician of amount spilled.	Y	N
COMMENTS:		

Evaluator_____

NAME _____

UNIT _____

DATE _____

COMPETENCY: Assisting With Exchange Transfusion (NICU)		
PERFORMANCE CRITERIA	**COMPLETED BY STAFF**	
1. Ascertains that MD or NNP have obtained appropriate informed consent has been signed.	Y	N
2. Notifies blood bank regarding indication for exchange.	Y	N
3. Ascertains that type and cross match have been done.	Y	N
4. Assembles equipment per unit procedure protocol, maintaining, sterile technique.	Y	N
5. Obtains correct patient's blood from blood bank.	Y	N
6. Prepares blood per unit procedure/protocol.	Y	N
7. Prepares infant per unit procedure/protocol.	Y	N
8. Administers albumin, if ordered.	Y	N
9. Sends initial withdrawn blood to lab per unit protocol.	Y	N
10. Initiates and maintains exchange record throughout procedure per unit protocol.	Y	N
11. Continuously monitors infant throughout procedure per unit protocol.	Y	N
12. Agitates blood bag *gently* every 10-15 minutes.	Y	N
13. Saves the last specimen withdrawn for further analysis per unit protocol.	Y	N
COMMENTS:		

Evaluator_____

NAME _____

UNIT _____

DATE _____

COMPETENCY: Chest Tube Maintenance (NICU)		
PERFORMANCE CRITERIA	**COMPLETED BY STAFF**	
1. Maintains security of tube connections with tape.	Y	N
2. Prevents tubing obstruction through kinking or other mechanical obstructions.	Y	N
3. Places and maintains drainage system below chest level.	Y	N
4. Maintains ordered water seal level in suction control chamber.	Y	N
5. Checks for bubbling in water seal chamber.	Y	N
6. Checks for gentle bubbling in the suction control chamber.	Y	N
7. Marks level of drainage collected in chest drainage unit.	Y	N
8. Milks chest tubes every hour.	Y	N
9. Documents according to unit standards.	Y	N
COMMENTS:		

Evaluator_____

135

NAME   _____

UNIT   _____

DATE   _____

COMPETENCY: Maintenance of Chest Tubes/Water-Seal Chest Drainage		
PERFORMANCE CRITERIA	**COMPLETED BY STAFF**	
1. Assesses site for bleeding, redness, swelling, heat, induration and drainage.	Y	N
2. Assesses for leakagbe of air or fluid around tube.	Y	N
3. Assesses patient for presence of respiratory distress and/or chest pain and reports immediately to physician if present.	Y	N
4. Checks tube connections and maintains secure attachment.	Y	N
5. Assesses drainage system for amount and charater of drainage and marks increments.	Y	N
6. Assesses drainage system for presence of blood or air.	Y	N
7. Checks tubing for obstructions and cleans it p.r.n.	Y	N
8. Assists patient with ROM exercises at least every 4 hrs. while awake on affected arm and shoulder.	Y	N
9. Assists patient with deep breathing/coughing every 2 hrs.	Y	N
10. Maintains air-tight drainage system in stabilized location below chest level.	Y	N
COMMENTS:		

Evaluator_____

NAME _____

UNIT _____

DATE _____

COMPETENCY: Scrubbing for Laparoscopic Cholecystectomy Procedures		
PERFORMANCE CRITERIA	**COMPLETED BY STAFF**	
1. Sets-up room equipment, supplies and instruments according to unit standards.	Y	N
2. Identifies instruments by name.	Y	N
3. Maintains sterile technique throughout procedure.	Y	N
4. Counts instruments at the designated times.	Y	N
5. Disposes of equipment and supplies appropriately.	Y	N
COMMENTS:		

Evaluator_____

NAME _____

UNIT _____

DATE _____

COMPETENCY: Circulating on Laparoscopic Cholecystectomy		
PERFORMANCE CRITERIA	**COMPLETED BY STAFF**	
1. Sets up room and equipment appropriately.	Y	N
2. Connects all tubing and light source correctly.	Y	N
3. Drapes video camera appropriately.	Y	N
4. Ensures that all equipment functions properly prior to procedure.	Y	N
5. Pre-sets insufflator prior to procedure.	Y	N
6. Pads patient's bony prominences.	Y	N
7. Maintains proper body alignment for patient.	Y	N
8. Completes charge slips, pharmacy requisitions and pathology information slips.	Y	N
COMMENTS:		

Evaluator_____

NAME   _____
UNIT   _____
DATE   _____

COMPETENCY: Circulating on Operative Procedure via Laser		
PERFORMANCE CRITERIA	**COMPLETED BY STAFF**	
1. Sets up room and equipment appropriately according to unit standards for Laser Procedures.	Y	N
2. Connects all tubing and light sources correctly.	Y	N
3. Drapes video camera appropriately prior to procedure.	Y	N
4. Ensures that all equipment functions properly prior to procedure.	Y	N
5. Pads patient's bony prominences.	Y	N
6. Maintains proper body alignment of patient before and during procedure.	Y	N
7. Documents all safety precautions on the Laser Checklist.	Y	N
8. Completes charge slips, pharmacy requisitions and pathology information slips.	Y	N
9. Cleans and stores equipment properly after each case.	Y	N
COMMENTS:		

Evaluator_____

NAME _____

UNIT _____

DATE _____

COMPETENCY: Collecting a Clean-Catch Urine Specimen		
PERFORMANCE CRITERIA	**COMPLETED BY STAFF**	
1. Provides specimen container to patient, labeled appropriately.	Y	N
2. Explains how to collect specimen to patient.	Y	N
3. Accepts specimen container from patient with gloves on.	Y	N
4. Confirms that specimen is labeled appropriately.	Y	N
5. Confirms that appropriate requisitions are attached to specimen.	Y	N
6. Places specimen and lab specimens into transport, maintaining universal precautions.	Y	N
7. Ensures that specimen is transported to the lab according to unit standards.	Y	N
COMMENTS:		

Evaluator_____

NAME _____

UNIT _____

DATE _____

COMPETENCY: Cleaning of Flexible Endoscopes		
PERFORMANCE CRITERIA	**COMPLETED BY STAFF**	
1. Washes hands and puts on non-sterile gloves.	Y	N
2. Disassembles scope properly.	Y	N
3. Cleans internal lumen of scope properly with peroxide, protozyme and water.	Y	N
4. Cleans external surface properly.	Y	N
5. Soaks scope in approved disinfectant for 20 minutes.	Y	N
6. Dries scope and replaces it in storage place identified by unit.	Y	N
COMMENTS:		

Evaluator_____

NAME _____

UNIT _____

DATE _____

COMPETENCY: Whirlpool Cleansing		
PERFORMANCE CRITERIA	**COMPLETED**	
	BY STAFF	
1. Fills tub to maximum height-water should fall below drain.	Y	N
2. Adds appropriate solution to water.	Y	N
3. Turns turbine on for 7-10 minutes.	Y	N
4. Scrubs tub with tub brush.	Y	N
5. Drains tub water.	Y	N
6. Rinses tub with clean running water.	Y	N
7. Sprays tub with alcohol.	Y	N
8. Rinses tub with clean water.	Y	N
COMMENTS:		

Evaluator_____

NAME   _____

UNIT   _____

DATE   _____

COMPETENCY: Clerical Support for Programs/Presentations		
PERFORMANCE CRITERIA	COMPLETED BY STAFF	
1. Schedule room, A-V and set-up.	Y	N
2. Notify staff of offering.	Y	N
3. Register staff for offering.	Y	N
4. Type handouts.	Y	N
5. Duplicate handouts.	Y	N
6. Generate transparencies.	Y	N
7. Collate packets if needed.	Y	N
8. Troubleshoot issues that may arise the day of program.	Y	N
COMMENTS:		

Evaluator_____

NAME   _____

UNIT   _____

DATE   _____

COMPETENCY: Utilization of Continuous Passive Motion (CPM) Machine	
PERFORMANCE CRITERIA	**COMPLETED BY STAFF**
1. When *applying*: validates correct patient.	Y N
2. Applies sheep skin to extremity.	Y N
3. Supports leg correctly while putting in CPM.	Y N
4. Validates correct knee-hip alignment.	Y N
5. Validates that CPM is in *extension* mode.	Y N
6. Turns CPM on.	Y N
7. Monitors for correct CPM function.	Y N
8. Monitors patient tolerance to procedure.	Y N
9. When *removing*: validates CPM in *extension* mode.	Y N
10. Validates proper patient position.	Y N
11. Turns off CPM.	Y N
12. Supports leg correctly while removing it from CPM.	Y N
13. Slowly lowers leg to bed.	Y N
COMMENTS:	

Evaluator_____

NAME _____

UNIT _____

DATE _____

COMPETENCY: Coordination of Educational Program		
PERFORMANCE CRITERIA	**COMPLETED** **BY STAFF**	
1. Identifies topic, audience and speakers.	Y	N
2. Identifies time frame for program.	Y	N
3. Arranges for room with appropriate set-up.	Y	N
4. Coordinates registration for the program.	Y	N
5. Identifies speaker(s) needs:		
a. A-V equipment	Y	N
b. parking	Y	N
c. duplication of materials	Y	N
6. Prepares program package including:		
a. objectives	Y	N
b. course content	Y	N
c. references	Y	N
d. handouts	Y	N
e. evaluation	Y	N
7. Reviews with speaker(s) any needs prior to program.		
8. Analyzes evaluations.		
9. Reports outcomes of program to appropriate sponsor.		
COMMENTS:		

Evaluator_____

NAME _____

UNIT _____

DATE _____

COMPETENCY: Project Management Coordination		
PERFORMANCE CRITERIA	**COMPLETED BY STAFF**	
1. Accepts responsibility for project management.	Y	N
2. Identifies appropriate team members.	Y	N
3. Schedules meetings and rooms.	Y	N
4. Sends agenda prior to meeting(s).	Y	N
5. Conducts meeting with productive outcomes.	Y	N
6. Arranges for minutes to be distributed within 5 days after meeting.	Y	N
7. Reports outcomes of project to appropriate sponsor.	Y	N
COMMENTS:		

Evaluator_____

NAME _____

UNIT _____

DATE _____

COMPETENCY: CT Verification/Documentation of Blood Work		
PERFORMANCE CRITERIA	**COMPLETED BY STAFF**	
1. Checks blood work prior to exam.	Y	N
2. Insures blood work is done within time period specified by department policy.	Y	N
3. Consults with Radiologist regarding patients with abnormal values.	Y	N
4. Documents blood work.	Y	N
5. Documents reason why IV contrast was not administered.	Y	N
6. Educates patient regarding exam and reason for blood work.	Y	N
7. Documents patient education.	Y	N
COMMENTS:		

Evaluator_____

NAME _____

UNIT _____

DATE _____

COMPETENCY: Crutch training	
PERFORMANCE CRITERIA	**COMPLETED BY STAFF**
1. Receives referral from Doctor with specifications.	Y N
2. Gets appropriate equipment based on referral i.e. walker, cane or crutches.	Y N
3. Receives weight or non-weight bearing status from referral.	Y N
4. Follows written directions from Doctor's referral.	Y N
5. Observes patient's ability to safely walk with equipment including steps, sitting and walking.	Y N
6. Initials referral for verification.	Y N
COMMENTS:	

Evaluator_____

148

NAME _____

UNIT _____

DATE _____

COMPETENCY: CVA Evaluation		
PERFORMANCE CRITERIA	**COMPLETED BY STAFF**	
1. Puts patient's name on the evaluation.	Y	N
2. Records date of evaluation.	Y	N
3. Records medical history.	Y	N
4. Defines expressive language skill level.	Y	N
5. Defines receptive language skill level.	Y	N
6. Evaluates oral/motor skills.	Y	N
7. Documents writing skills.	Y	N
8. Documents reading skills.	Y	N
9. Documents impressions with severity level noted.	Y	N
10. Documents short term goals.	Y	N
11. Documents long term goals.	Y	N
12. Documents Rehab potential.	Y	N
COMMENTS:		

Evaluator_____

NAME _____

UNIT _____

DATE _____

COMPETENCY: Defibrillation		
PERFORMANCE CRITERIA	COMPLETED BY STAFF	
1. Assess lead placement.	Y	N
2. Assesses and identifies signs and symptoms of fibrillation including unresponsiveness, pulselessness, or ECG showing V-tach, V-fib.	Y	N
3. Gathers appropriate equipment/supplies for defibrillation.	Y	N
4. Plugs in equipment with appropriate grounding source. Turns power on.	Y	N
5. Prepares defibrillator paddles - covers paddles with either conductive pads or gel.	Y	N
6. Places paddles in correct position either: a. 1 paddle in 2nd intercostal space just to right of sternum and 1 paddle under left nipple OR b. 1 paddle left interscapular area and 1 paddle at 3rd intercostal space	Y	N
7. Quick-checks rhythm to assure presence of fibrillation, and V-tach.	Y	N
8. Adjust watt-second dial in the following sequence (dependent of rhythm): a. Initial attempt: 200 joules b. 2nd attempt: 300 joules c. 3rd and successive attempts: 360 joules	Y	N
9. Assesses that defibrillator is in the asynchronous mode and rechecks rhythm.	Y	N
10. Yells "CLEAR" loudly and waits for all ancillary personnel to back away from patient.	Y	N
11. Depresses the discharge buttons on both paddles with 20 to 25 lbs. of pressure against chest wall until current is delivered. Make sure 100% surface contact is made.	Y	N
12. Rechecks rhythm. If fibrillation is still present, restarts sequences 6 to 10 pausing to recharge paddles to appropriate level of joules, per physician order.	Y	N
COMMENTS: Type of Equipment: _____ _____		

Evaluator_____

NAME _____
UNIT _____
DATE _____

COMPETENCY: Delegating Work Assignments		
PERFORMANCE CRITERIA	**COMPLETED BY STAFF**	
1. Identifies work to be completed.	Y	N
2. Chooses appropriate staff member to complete identified work, according to job descriptions.	Y	N
3. Develops equitable work assignments based on the scope of work identified.	Y	N
4. Clearly communicates work assignments.	Y	N
5. Clearly explains prioritization of work assignments.	Y	N
6. Clearly establishes communication check points.	Y	N
7. Defines time limitations for completion of work.	Y	N
8. Provides feedback concerning quality of work.	Y	N
COMMENTS:		

Evaluator_____

NAME   _____

UNIT   _____

DATE   _____

COMPETENCY: Correction of Diabetic Menus		
PERFORMANCE CRITERIA	**COMPLETED BY STAFF**	
1. Diet pattern is accurate.	Y	N
2. Menu selection is consistent with diet pattern.	Y	N
3. Alteration in diet pattern is appropriate.	Y	N
4. Portion sizes are written appropriately.	Y	N
5. Menu is legible for trayline.	Y	N
6. Menu is highlighted accurately.	Y	N
COMMENTS:		

Evaluator_____

NAME _____
UNIT _____
DATE _____

COMPETENCY: Providing Diabetic Teaching		
PERFORMANCE CRITERIA	COMPLETED BY STAFF	
1. Verifies physician referral for diabetic teaching.	Y	N
2. Assesses patient/family for knowledge base.	Y	N
3. Provides diabetic teaching according to unit standard.	Y	N
4. Assessess patient learning.	Y	N
5. Reinforces information p.r.n.	Y	N
6. Provides appropriate written literature.	Y	N
7. Provides patient with the telephone number of a contact person/resource individual.	Y	N
8. Documents patient teaching.	Y	N
COMMENTS:		

Evaluator_____

NAME   _____

UNIT   _____

DATE   _____

COMPETENCY: Peritoneal Dialysis Exchange Procedure		
PERFORMANCE CRITERIA	COMPLETED BY STAFF	
1. Gathers all appropriate supplies.	Y	N
2. Prepares solution bag per physician order.	Y	N
3. Properly connects solution bag to peritoneal catheter.	Y	N
4. Flushes drain bag appropriately.	Y	N
5. Completely drains dialysis solution.	Y	N
6. Slowly infuses solution.	Y	N
7. Completely closes peritoneal clamp.	Y	N
8. Properly disconnects empty solution bag from peritoneal catheter.	Y	N
9. Properly disposes of peritoneal drainage.	Y	N
COMMENTS:		

Evaluator_____

NAME _____
UNIT _____
DATE _____

COMPETENCY: Setting Up Diet Trays and Assisting Patients in Eating		
PERFORMANCE CRITERIA	**COMPLETED BY STAFF**	
1. Assists patient into sitting position and covers chest with towel.	Y	N
2. Washes hands of patient and care provider.	Y	N
3. Ensures that the tray is labeled with the correct patient's name.	Y	N
4. Assists patient to identify food types on tray.	Y	N
5. Using spoon only, offers small portions of food to patient. Ensures that patient has swallowed portion before offering another.	Y	N
6. Reminds patient of hot or cold temperatures when offering a different food.	Y	N
7. Alternates fluids and solids throughout meal.	Y	N
8. Encourages patient to eat independently within the patient's limitations.	Y	N
9. Cleans tray, patient and bed following the meal.	Y	N
10. Documents intake as appropriate.	Y	N
11. Notifies RN of patient's inability to swallow food or difficulty in eating.	Y	N
COMMENTS:		

Evaluator_____

NAME   _____

UNIT   _____

DATE   _____

COMPETENCY: Discharge Report Dictation		
PERFORMANCE CRITERIA	COMPLETED BY STAFF	
1. Gives patient's name.	Y	N
2. Gives medical record number.	Y	N
3. Gives referring physician.	Y	N
4. Gives date of original evaluation.	Y	N
5. States patient's progress.	Y	N
6. States patient's present status in therapy.	Y	N
7. States discharge plans.	Y	N
COMMENTS:		

Evaluator_____

NAME   _____

UNIT   _____

DATE   _____

COMPETENCY: Medical Record Documentation (In-Patient) of Nutritional Evaluation		
PERFORMANCE CRITERIA	**COMPLETED BY STAFF**	
1. The following information is written in the initial Nutrition Note in the Medical Record:		
a. appropriate subjective data	Y	N
b. accurate objective data including:		
1. diagnosis	Y	N
2. height	Y	N
3. weight	Y	N
4. pertinent laboratory data	Y	N
5. pertinent medications	Y	N
6. pertinent diagnostic test results	Y	N
7. diet order	Y	N
c. accurate assessment data including:		
1. diet history	Y	N
2. current intake	Y	N
3. tolerance to nutritional therapy	Y	N
4. analysis of pertinent laboratory data	Y	N
5. appropriateness of the diet	Y	N
6. degree of nutritional risk	Y	N
7. need for education	Y	N
d. appropriate plans	Y	N
2. Documents in black ink.	Y	N
3. Heads the note with date.	Y	N
4. Heads the note with Nutrition Note.	Y	N
5. Heads the note with time of day.	Y	N
6. Signs note with signature and credentials.	Y	N
COMMENTS:		

Evaluator_____

157

NAME _____

UNIT _____

DATE _____

COMPETENCY: Medical Record Documentation (Out-patient) of Nutritional Evaluation		
PERFORMANCE CRITERIA	**COMPLETED BY STAFF**	
1. The following information is written in the initial Nutrition Note on the designated Nutrition Form.		
a. referring physician or clinic	Y	N
b. today's date	Y	N
c. reason for consult	Y	N
d. appropriate subjective data including:	Y	N
1. usual weight at 25 years of age	Y	N
2. physical activity	Y	N
e. accurate objective data including:	Y	N
1. age	Y	N
2. height	Y	N
3. weight	Y	N
4. reasonable body weight	Y	N
5. estimated needs for weight maintenance	Y	N
6. pertinent labs	Y	N
7. pertinent medications	Y	N
8. nutrition therapy/counseling provided	Y	N
f. accurate assessment data including:	Y	N
1. percent of reasonable body weight	Y	N
2. diet history	Y	N
3. comprehension of counseling	Y	N
4. adherence to suggestions	Y	N
g. appropriate plans	Y	N
2. Documents in black ink.	Y	N
3. Signs note with signature and credentials.	Y	N
COMMENTS:		

Evaluator_____

158

NAME   _____

UNIT   _____

DATE   _____

COMPETENCY: Dressing Change After Whirlpool Treatment		
PERFORMANCE CRITERIA	**COMPLETED BY STAFF**	
1. Unwraps original dressing from wound.	Y	N
2. Places wound in whirlpool for 20 minutes.	Y	N
3. Removes wound from whirlpool.	Y	N

4. Uses appropriate techniques for dressing.
    a. debredes wound
    b. applies solution (i.e. wet-dry, normal saline, silvadine, or
       duoderm)
	Y	N

5. Wraps wound according to doctor's orders.	Y	N
COMMENTS:		

Evaluator_____

NAME   _____

UNIT   _____

DATE   _____

COMPETENCY: Perform Echocardiogram/Doppler		
PERFORMANCE CRITERIA	COMPLETED BY STAFF	
1. Instructs patient about test.	Y	N
2. Puts patient information into machine.	Y	N
3. Checks VCR tape for proper set up.	Y	N
4. Places patient on left side.	Y	N
5. Places transducer on chest in appropriate area to best see heart structures.	Y	N
6. Records all information.	Y	N
7. Cleans patient when finished.	Y	N
8. Measures and prepares Echo for physician to read.	Y	N
9. Sends report to patient's physician.	Y	N
10. Charts patient information on log.	Y	N
COMMENTS:		

Evaluator_____

NAME   _____

UNIT   _____

DATE   _____

COMPETENCY: Perform Pediatric Echocardiogram/Doppler		
PERFORMANCE CRITERIA	**COMPLETED**	**BY STAFF**
1. Puts patient information into machine.	Y	N
2. Checks VCR tape for proper set up.	Y	N
3. Scrubs and gowns.	Y	N
4. Preps infant or child.	Y	N
5. Puts infant or child in proper position as indicated.	Y	N
6. Places tracsducer on chest in appropriate area to best see heart structures.	Y	N
7. Records all information.	Y	N
8. Takes measurements while recording.	Y	N
9. Cleans patient when finished.	Y	N
10. Charts patient information on logs.	Y	N
COMMENTS:		

Evaluator_____

NAME   _____

UNIT   _____

DATE   _____

COMPETENCY: 12 Lead ECG Placement		
PERFORMANCE CRITERIA	**COMPLETED BY STAFF**	
1. Prepares patient by placing patient in a comfortable, slightly elevated position.	Y	N
2. Checks that patient is not touching any metal part of bed.	Y	N
3. Applies clean electrodes to extremities.	Y	N
4. Connects cable to electrodes on patient extremities: a. RA (white) to right arm b. LA (black) to left arm c. RL (green) to right leg d. LL (red) to left leg	Y	N
5. Places electrodes and cables to chest wall: a: V_1: 4th intercostal space to right of sternum b. V_2: 4th intercostal space to left of sternum c. V_3: midway between V_2 and V_4 d. V_4: at 5th intercostal space mid-clavicular line e. V_5: at 5th intercostal space anterior axillary line f. V_6: at 5th intercostal space mid-axillary line	Y	N
COMMENTS:		

Evaluator_____

NAME _____

UNIT _____

DATE _____

COMPETENCY: 12 Lead ECG Preparation		
PERFORMANCE CRITERIA	**COMPLETED BY STAFF**	
1. Explains to patient that ECG will be obtained.	Y	N
2. Prepares patient by placing patient in a comfortable, slightly elevated position.	Y	N
3. Checks that patient is not touching any metal part of bed.	Y	N
4. Preps skin.	Y	N
5. Applies clean electrodes to extremities.	Y	N
6. Connects cable to electrodes on patient extremities: a. RA (white) to right arm b. LA (black) to left arm c. RL (green) to right leg d. LL (red) to left leg	Y	N
7. Places electrodes and cables to chest wall: a: V_1: 4th intercostal space to right of sternum b. V_2: 4th intercostal space to left of sternum c. V_3: midway between V_2 and V_4 d. V_4: at 5th intercostal space mid-clavicular line e. V_5: at 5th intercostal space anterior axillary line f. V_6: at 5th intercostal space mid-axillary line	Y	N
COMMENTS:		

Evaluator_____

NAME _____

UNIT _____

DATE _____

COMPETENCY: Performs Electrocardiogram		
PERFORMANCE CRITERIA	COMPLETED BY STAFF	
1. Instructs patients about test.	Y	N
2. Places electrodes on patient carefully to insure proper positioning.	Y	N
3. Records patient information on EKG machine.	Y	N
4. Attaches leads to electrodes.	Y	N
5. Reviews EKG tracing during test.	Y	N
6. Prepares tracings for Doctor to read.	Y	N
COMMENTS:		

Evaluator_____

NAME _____

UNIT _____

DATE _____

COMPETENCY: Performs Electrocardiogram on Marquette		
PERFORMANCE CRITERIA	**COMPLETED BY STAFF**	
1. Instructs patients about test.	Y	N
2. Preps patients according to department protocol.	Y	N
3. Records tracing according to department protocol.	Y	N
4. Prepares tracing for physician to read.	Y	N
5. Charts in-patient confirmed EKG's according to department procedures.	Y	N
COMMENTS:		

Evaluator_____

NAME _____

UNIT _____

DATE _____

COMPETENCY: Obtaining 12 Lead ECG - Marquette Machine		
PERFORMANCE CRITERIA	**COMPLETED BY STAFF**	
1. Instructs patient regarding test to be performed.	Y	N
2. Plugs in machines and turn on.	Y	N
3. Puts in required patient information.	Y	N
4. Prepares patient as per Preparation Criteria.	Y	N
5. Ensures paper in machine.	Y	N
6. Pushes 12 Lead button.	Y	N
7. Observes strip for good quality.	Y	N
8. Saves information to disc.	Y	N
9. Removes equipment from patient.	Y	N
10. Cleans skin.	Y	N
11. If an in-patient, place copy of unconfirmed tracing on In-patient Chart.	Y	N
12. Prepares tracing for Cardiologist to read according to department procedures.	Y	N
13. Ensures confirmed copy charted or sent to physician.	Y	N
COMMENTS:		

Evaluator_____

NAME   _____

UNIT   _____

DATE   _____

COMPETENCY: Obtaining 12 Lead ECG - Pagewriter		
PERFORMANCE CRITERIA	**COMPLETED BY STAFF**	
1. Plugs in machine and turns switch to "on" position.	Y	N
2. Explains to patient that ECG will be obtained.	Y	N
3. Turns format switch to "2".	Y	N

4.   Places electrodes in appropriate positions:
   a. Left leg
   b. Right leg
   c. Left arm
   d. Right arm
   e. V_1: 4th intercostal space to right of sternum
   f. V_2: 4th intercostal space to left of sternum
   g. V_3: midway between V_2 and V_4
   h. V_4: at 5th intercostal space mid-clavicular line
   i. V_5: at 5th intercostal space anterior axillary line
   j. V_6: at 5th intercostal space mid-axillary line
	Y	N

5. Places paper in ready position and pushes "auto" button to begin ECG	Y	N
6. Writes patient's name and room number on top of ECG paper upon completion.	Y	N
7. Obtains copy of ECG by pushing "copy" button.	Y	N
8. Removes all lead and reorganizes equipment on ECG cart.	Y	N
COMMENTS:		

Evaluator_____

NAME _____

UNIT _____

DATE _____

COMPETENCY: Application of Electronic Fetal Monitor (External)		
PERFORMANCE CRITERIA	**COMPLETED BY STAFF**	
1. Explains procedure and purpose of EFM to patient and family.	Y	N
2. Plugs tocodynamometer and ultrasound transducer into correct outlets.	Y	N
3. Places tocodynamometer in correct position for gestational age.	Y	N
4. Places ultrasound transducer over fetal back, using appropriate amount of transducer gel.	Y	N
5. Validates accuracy of uterine activity printout.	Y	N
6. Validates that fetal heart rate is the FHR and NOT the maternal heart rate.	Y	N
7. Applies belts to tocodynamometer and transducer without effecting the accuracy of EFM data.	Y	N
8. Rests tocodynamometer to appropriate resting tone.	Y	N
9. Positions patient to obtain the most accurate and clear data pattern (LLP).	Y	N
10. Labels EFM strip correctly and legibly.	Y	N
COMMENTS:		

Evaluator_____

NAME   _____

UNIT   _____

DATE   _____

COMPETENCY: Obtaining 30 Minute EFM		
PERFORMANCE CRITERIA	**COMPLETED BY STAFF**	
1. Verifies fetal heart rate as that of fetus.	Y	N
2. Sets uterine resting tone within allowed range.	Y	N
3. Positions patient in LLT or LLP.	Y	N
4. Relocates ultrasound until continuous FHR tracing is obtained.	Y	N
5. Records on strip any patient care interventions completed.	Y	N
6. Records on strip maternal activity.	Y	N
7. Checks strip twice during 30 minute period for continuity of FHR tracing.	Y	N
8. Relocates ultrasound if non-continuous FHR tracing is present.	Y	N
9. At end of 30 minute strip, signs off on strip.	Y	N
COMMENTS:		

Evaluator_____

NAME _____

UNIT _____

DATE _____

COMPETENCY: Interpretation of Electronic Fetal Monitor (External)		
PERFORMANCE CRITERIA	COMPLETED BY STAFF	
1. Distinguishes between uterine activity, FHR activity and artifact.	Y	N
2. Interprets uterine activity correctly.	Y	N
3. Identifies baseline FHR and determines whether it is normal or abnormal.	Y	N
4. Determine whether periodic FHR changes are normal/abnormal.	Y	N
5. Initiates appropriate corrective action for abnormal FHR patterns and/or uterine activity.	Y	N
6. Documents actions on strip, legibly.	Y	N
7. Notifies physician appropriately for abnormal EFM data.	Y	N
8. Explains data to patient and family.	Y	N
9. Correctly documents EFM data in nurses' notes.	Y	N
COMMENTS:		

Evaluator_____

NAME _____
UNIT _____
DATE _____

COMPETENCY: Recognition of Selected Fetal Monitoring Patterns		
PERFORMANCE CRITERIA	COMPLETED BY STAFF	
1. Identifies baseline fetal heart rate.	Y	N
2. Determines whether fetal heart rate baseline is normal.	Y	N
3. Identifies uterine activity status.	Y	N
4. Identifies periodic fetal heart rate patterns.	Y	N
5. States whether periodic fetal heart rate pattern ominous.	Y	N
6. Implements patient care intervention(s) appropriately for demonstrated periodic patterns.	Y	N
7. Reports non-reassuring fetal heart rate patterns on baseline to appropriate personnel.	Y	N
8. Identifies uterine activity which places maternal and/or fetal health at risk.	Y	N
9. Identifies variations in uterine activity which do not require interventions.	Y	N
10. Identifies reassuring fetal heart rate pattern(s) and baseline.	Y	N
COMMENTS:		

Evaluator_____

NAME _____

UNIT _____

DATE _____

COMPETENCY: Setting Up Continuous Enteral Tubing Feedings		
PERFORMANCE CRITERIA	**COMPLETED BY STAFF**	
1. Validates correct formula for patient.	Y	N
2. Validates that feeding is being set-up for correct patient.	Y	N
3. Ensures that formula is at room temperature.	Y	N
4. Shakes formula container prior to placing in feeding bag.	Y	N
5. Pours formula into feeding bag with clamp closed.	Y	N
6. Hangs formula on infusion pump.	Y	N
7. Primes tubing so that all air is purged.	Y	N
8. Plugs pump into electrical outlet.	Y	N
9. Notifies nurse that feeding is ready to be initiated.	Y	N
COMMENTS:		

Evaluator_____

172

NAME   _____

UNIT   _____

DATE   _____

COMPETENCY: Utilization of ERCP Equipment		
PERFORMANCE CRITERIA	**COMPLETED BY STAFF**	
1. Assembles ERCP equipment.	Y	N
2. Identifies ERCP equipment by name.	Y	N
3. Hand appropriate equipment to physician as requested.	Y	N
4. Maintains clean techniques throughout procedure.	Y	N
5. Disposes of equipment properly.	Y	N
COMMENTS:		

Evaluator_____

NAME _____

UNIT _____

DATE _____

COMPETENCY: Employee Counseling for Performance Related Issues		
PERFORMANCE CRITERIA	**COMPLETED**	
	BY STAFF	
1. Identifies performance issue.	Y	N
2. Gathers data (anecdotals, direct observation, peer review, etc.) related to the issue.	Y	N
3. Schedules counseling appointment with employee.	Y	N
4. Provide private location for counseling session.	Y	N
5. Identifies performance issue with employee.	Y	N
6. Reviews data with employee.	Y	N
7. Solicits employee response/feedback on issue.	Y	N
8. Collaboratively formulates action plan with employee to improve the employee's performance.	Y	N
9. Documents action plan.	Y	N
10. Obtains employee's signature on action plan.	Y	N
11. Provides copy of action plan to: a. employee b. employee's personnel file	Y	N
12. Reviews employee's performance for determination of improvement related to issue in action plan.	Y	N
13. Provides verbal feedback to employee related to performance issue within 1 week.	Y	N
COMMENTS:		

Evaluator_____

174

NAME   _____

UNIT   _____

DATE   _____

COMPETENCY: **Complying with Legal Requirements for the Newly Hired Employee**		
PERFORMANCE CRITERIA	COMPLETED BY STAFF	
1. Completes and/or updates job description with ADA regulations and job performance standards prior to posting or advertising of job.	Y	N
2. Reviews two documents to prove candidate's identity and right to work (ie. Social Security Card, US Birth Certificate, Drivers License, Government ID Card, etc.) prior to employment offer.	Y	N
3. Ascertains favorable reference check prior to scheduling physical and offer of employment.	Y	N
4. Ascertains that candidate has passed physical and drug screen prior to offer of employment.	Y	N
COMMENTS:		

Evaluator_____

NAME   _____

UNIT   _____

DATE   _____

COMPETENCY: Reviews Employee Radiation Dosimetry Report		
PERFORMANCE CRITERIA	**COMPLETED BY STAFF**	
1. Reviews monthly dosimetry report for employee exposure.	Y	N
a. Identifies individuals whose readings are close to or above action levels.	Y	N
b. Identifies the reason for high reading.	Y	N
c. Date and sign report.	Y	N
d. Reports findings to the department.	Y	N
e. Posts report in the department.	Y	N
f. Remediates staff with action levels.	Y	N
2. Manages facility exposure.	Y	N
a. Maintains daily record of radiopharmaceuticals and sealed sources.	Y	N
b. Maintains daily record of department exposure (wipes, surveys, etc.)	Y	N
c. Evaluates daily records for unacceptable readings.	Y	N
d. Documents action taken by the department for unacceptable levels.	Y	N
COMMENTS:		

Evaluator_____

NAME _____

UNIT _____

DATE _____

COMPETENCY: Entering an Isolation Room		
PERFORMANCE CRITERIA	**COMPLETED BY STAFF**	
1. Identifies specific isolation techniques required.	Y	N
2. Washes hands thoroughly.	Y	N

3. Correctly puts on gown if indicated:
   a. puts gown on with opening in the back
   b. fastens neck band
   c. fastens back tie, completely covering clothes/uniform
	Y	N

4. Correctly puts on mask if indicated:
   a. places mask over nose and mouth touching only the strings
   b. ties top strings over ears
   c. ties lower strings
	Y	N

5. Correctly applies gloves if indicated:
   a. chooses appropriate glove type
   b. puts on gloves (using sterile technique for sterile gloves)
   c. ensures that glove covers isolation wrist band
	Y	N

COMMENTS:		

Evaluator_____

NAME   _____

UNIT   _____

DATE   _____

COMPETENCY: Extubation		
PERFORMANCE CRITERIA	**COMPLETED BY STAFF**	
1. Verifies written order for removal of Endotracheal Tube.	Y	N
2. Assesses patient for: a. stable respiratory rate and volume b. adequate muscle strength (via head lift and hand grip)	Y	N
3. Assembles appropriate equipment per unit standard.	Y	N
4. Places patient in semi-fowler position.	Y	N
5. Uses aseptic technique to insert suction catheter deep into Endotracheal Tube.	Y	N
6. Suctions all secretions using no more than 15 seconds to suction at a time.	Y	N
7. Ensures no secretions above the cuff via suctioning oral cavity according to unit standards.	Y	N
8. Deflates cuff on ET Tube.	Y	N
9. Gently removes ET Tube maintaining sterile techniques.	Y	N
10. Suctions trachea prn during ET Tube removal according to unit standards.	Y	N
11. Observes patient for signs of respiratory distress or difficulty, tachycardia, diaphoresis.	Y	N
12. Immediately starts O_2 Therapy.	Y	N
13. Accurately checks O_2 Saturation throughout O_2 Therapy.	Y	N
14. Documents actions and patient response.	Y	N
COMMENTS:		

Evaluator_____

NAME   _____

UNIT   _____

DATE   _____

COMPETENCY: Fabricate & Issue a Dynamic Splint		
PERFORMANCE CRITERIA	**COMPLETED BY STAFF**	
1. Performs Musculoskeletal assessment.	Y	N
2. Determines the type of Dynamic Splint indicated.	Y	N
3. Develops a pattern for splint.	Y	N
4. Uses appropriate splint material.	Y	N
5. Safely heats splint material.	Y	N
6. Positions upper extremity.	Y	N
7. Applies splint material to extremity.	Y	N
8. Reposition upper extremity in splint.	Y	N
9. Applies Outrigger system to splint.	Y	N
10. Applies Dynamic Cuff to appendage.	Y	N
11. Applies Dynamic Cuff to appropriate angle of pull.	Y	N
12. Applies strapping.	Y	N
13. Checks for pressure areas.	Y	N
14. Provides patient with splint schedule.	Y	N
15. Instructs patient in splint precautions and care.	Y	N
COMMENTS:		

Evaluator_____

NAME _____

UNIT _____

DATE _____

COMPETENCY: Fabricate and Issue a Static Splint		
PERFORMANCE CRITERIA	**COMPLETED BY STAFF**	
1. Determines the type of splint indicated.	Y	N
2. Develops a pattern for splint.	Y	N
3. Uses appropriate splint material.	Y	N
4. Safely heats splint material.	Y	N
5. Positions upper extremity.	Y	N
6. Applies splint material to extremity.	Y	N
7. Repositions upper extremity in splint.	Y	N
8. Applies strapping.	Y	N
9. Checks for pressure areas.	Y	N
10. Provides patient with splint schedule.	Y	N
11. Instructs patient in splint precautions and care.	Y	N
COMMENTS:		

Evaluator_____

NAME   _____

UNIT   _____

DATE   _____

COMPETENCY: Flexes Staffing According to Census on a Shift-by-Shift Basis	
PERFORMANCE CRITERIA	COMPLETED BY STAFF
1. Ascertains patient census or volume statistic at least 2 hours prior to beginning of shift.	Y N
2. Ascertains acuity/severity data (if appropriate).	Y N
3. Projects human resource requirements to meet the staffing needs.	Y N
4. Compares scheduled staff to actual need, making a determination regarding variance of staff.	Y N

5. Flexes staffing appropriately:
  * Additional resources needed - calls per diem staff to come in - negotiates with staff to reschedule themselves to cover variance.
  * Staffing is appropriate for volume and acuity - no action needed.
  * Resources surpass staffing need - reschedules staff to remove surplus.
	Y N

COMMENTS:	

Evaluator_____

181

NAME _____

UNIT _____

DATE _____

COMPETENCY: Insertion of Foley Catheters		
PERFORMANCE CRITERIA	**COMPLETED BY STAFF**	
1. Provides privacy for patient and explains procedure.	Y	N
2. Positions and drapes patient appropriately.	Y	N
3. Opens catheter kit setting up sterile field.	Y	N
4. Dons sterile gloves and sets up catheter supplies.	Y	N
5. Tests catheter balloon for leaks and attaches it to drainage bag included in kit.	Y	N
6. Lubricates catheter tip with water soluble lubricant.	Y	N
7. Prepares periurethral area with sterile procedure.	Y	N
8. Gently inserts catheter to appropriate length.	Y	N
9. Validates correct placement by observing for urine flow through catheter tube.	Y	N
10. Inflates balloon with 6-10 cc of sterile water and retracts catheter gently until resistance is felt.	Y	N
11. Anchors catheter appropriately and hangs drainage bag on bed frame below patient's body.	Y	N
12. Reports to nurse the time of insertion, color and amount of urine and patient's tolerance to procedure.	Y	N
COMMENTS:		

Evaluator_____

NAME _____

UNIT _____

DATE _____

COMPETENCY: Maintenance of Gas Tank Gauges		
PERFORMANCE CRITERIA	**COMPLETED**	
	BY STAFF	
1. Assembles necessary equipment.	Y	N
2. Identifies appropriate gauges for each tank.	Y	N
3. Properly changes gauges.	Y	N
4. Appropriately disposes of equipment.	Y	N
COMMENTS:		

Evaluator_____

NAME _____

UNIT _____

DATE _____

COMPETENCY: Handwashing		
PERFORMANCE CRITERIA	**COMPLETED BY STAFF**	
1. Completely wets hands and wrists, with fingers pointed downward.	Y	N
2. Applies soap, spreading lather over entire area of hands and 2 inches above the wrists.	Y	N
3. Develops friction, rubbing vigorously for at least one minute.	Y	N
4. Rinses well with fingers pointed downward.	Y	N
5. Dries area completely with paper towels.	Y	N
6. Turns off faucet with a dry paper towel.	Y	N
COMMENTS:		

Evaluator_____

NAME   _____

UNIT   _____

DATE   _____

COMPETENCY: Care of Harmonic Scalpel		
PERFORMANCE CRITERIA	COMPLETED BY STAFF	
1. Identifies all disposable parts.	Y	N
2. Disconnects disposable parts.	Y	N
3. Appropriately disposes of single use parts.	Y	N
4. Disinfects disposable parts according to unit standards.	Y	N
5. Implements Terminal Sterilization according to unit standards.	Y	N
COMMENTS:		

Evaluator_____

NAME   _____

UNIT   _____

DATE   _____

COMPETENCY: Application of Holter Monitor		
PERFORMANCE CRITERIA	COMPLETED BY STAFF	
1. Instructs patient about tests.	Y	N
2. Preps skin thoroughly.	Y	N
3. Applies electrodes correctly.	Y	N
4. Attaches patient to monitor.	Y	N
5. Checks monitor for proper operation.	Y	N
6. Tapes leads to patient's chest.	Y	N
7. Explains diary sheet to patient.	Y	N
COMMENTS:		

Evaluator_____

NAME   _____

UNIT   _____

DATE   _____

COMPETENCY: Taking Infant Weights		
PERFORMANCE CRITERIA	**COMPLETED BY STAFF**	
1. Explains procedure to family	Y	N
2. Places clean liner on scale.	Y	N
3. Removes infant's clothing except for T-shirt and diaper.	Y	N
4. Places infant on scales.	Y	N
5. Identifies infant's weight as that weight which is the most constant.	Y	N
6. Immediately redresses infant after removing infant from scales.	Y	N
7. Subtracts weight of T-shirt and similar diaper from weight obtained.	Y	N
8. Documents appropriately.	Y	N
COMMENTS:		

Evaluator_____

NAME _____

UNIT _____

DATE _____

COMPETENCY: Infusion Pump Set-Up		
PERFORMANCE CRITERIA	**COMPLETED BY STAFF**	
1. Assembles appropriate equipment.	Y	N
2. Plugs in and turns on pump.	Y	N
3. Sets up IV using appropriate tubing and filters.	Y	N
4. Primes tubing and closes clamp.	Y	N
5. Inserts IV set into pump correctly.	Y	N
6. Sets rate and volume to be infused.	Y	N
7. Opens clamp and presses "start".	Y	N
COMMENTS:		

Evaluator_____

NAME   _____

UNIT   _____

DATE   _____

EQUIPMENT: _____

COMPETENCY: Instrument Maintenance		
PERFORMANCE CRITERIA	COMPLETED BY STAFF	
1. Performs instrument maintenance according to departmental policy and procedure.	Y	N
2. Trouble shoots functional errors to determine corrective action.	Y	N
3. Implements corrective action.	Y	N
4. Documents maintenance on appropriate form.	Y	N
5. Performs function check according to departmental procedure.	Y	N
6. Documents appropriately.	Y	N
COMMENTS:		

Evaluator_____

NAME   _____

UNIT   _____

DATE   _____

COMPETENCY: Administration of IV Push Medications		
PERFORMANCE CRITERIA	**COMPLETED BY STAFF**	
1. Checks written order for medication.	Y	N
2. Checks patient's chart for allergies.	Y	N
3. Prepares prescribed medication into appropriate syringe.	Y	N
4. Checks IV solution compatibility with medication to be given.	Y	N
5. Rechecks with patient, if possible, about allergies.	Y	N
6. Checks IV for patency.	Y	N
7. Clamps or pinches off IV tubing.	Y	N
8. Wipes off medicinal entry port with alcohol swab.	Y	N
9. Inserts needle into entry port and injects medication according to recommended IV push rate.	Y	N
10. Withdraws needle, unclamps IV tubing and rechecks IV flow rate.	Y	N
11. Monitors patient for adverse or untoward reactions.	Y	N
12. Disposes of needle and syringe in appropriate containers according to Structure Standards.	Y	N
COMMENTS:		

Evaluator_____

NAME _____

UNIT _____

DATE _____

COMPETENCY: Administration of IV Push Medications to Infants		
PERFORMANCE CRITERIA	**COMPLETED BY STAFF**	
1. Checks written order for medication.	Y	N
2. Checks patient's chart for allergies.	Y	N
3. Prepares prescribed medication into appropriate syringe.	Y	N
4. Checks patient ID bracelet.	Y	N
5. Flushes Heplock with 1.0 cc NS to check patency.	Y	N
6. Wipes off medicinal entry port with alcohol swab.	Y	N
7. Injects medicine slowly according to recommended IV Push rate for infants (see unit standards).	Y	N
8. After medication is completed, flushes with 1 cc NS, followed by 1 cc 10u/cc Heparin Flush.	Y	N
9. Monitors patient for adverse or untoward reactions.	Y	N
10. Disposes of needle and syringe in appropriate containers according to Structure Standards.	Y	N
COMMENTS:		

Evaluator_____

NAME   _____

UNIT   _____

DATE   _____

COMPETENCY: IV Conscious Sedation		
PERFORMANCE CRITERIA	**COMPLETED BY STAFF**	

1. Assesses for contraindication of conscious sedation including:
   a. O_2 Saturation < 90
   b. Diastolic BP > 120
   c. Presence of significant arrhythmia
	Y	N

2. Checks IV site for patency.	Y	N
3. Collects baseline Vital Signs.	Y	N
4. Administers medication per physician order/hospital policy.	Y	N

5. Monitors patient throughout procedure for:
   a. Significant change in Vital Signs
   b. Drop in O_2 Saturation
	Y	N

6. Notifies physician of changes or adverse reactions.	Y	N

7. Administers reversal agents as needed per physician order:
   a. Narcan for Demerol or Fentanyl
   b. Romazican for Versed
	Y	N

COMMENTS:		

Evaluator_____

NAME   _____

UNIT   _____

DATE   _____

COMPETENCY: Peripheral IV Insertion		
PERFORMANCE CRITERIA	COMPLETED BY STAFF	
1. Validates physician order. Explains procedure to patient and checks for allergies and presence of mastectomy.	Y	N
2. Chooses and assembles all appropriate equipment.	Y	N
3. Washes hands thoroughly.	Y	N
4. Selects appropriate site and catheter size. Applies tourniquet 2-3 inches above insertion site.	Y	N
5. Prepares site using alcohol, acetone and/or betadine swabsticks for at least 1 minute allowing site to air dry.	Y	N
6. Puts on non-sterile gloves.	Y	N
7. Performs venipuncture, inserting catheter with bevel up to 30 degree angle.	Y	N
8. Checks for blood return in catheter.	Y	N
9. Releases tourniquet and removes stylet.	Y	N
10. Flushes catheter with normal saline solution and attaches tubing or adapter to T-connector.	Y	N
11. Applies sterile dressing and labels dressing with date, time and gauge of catheter and initials of person inserting catheter. (Tegaderm for inpatients, 2x2 gauze or bandaid for outpatients).	Y	N
12. Secures catheter to limb.	Y	N
13. Disposes of venipuncture equipment in appropriate containers according to Safety Standards.	Y	N
14. Educates patient concerning purpose and need for IV therapy.	Y	N
COMMENTS:		

Evaluator_____

NAME _____

UNIT _____

DATE _____

COMPETENCY: Discontinuation of Peripheral IV Infusion		
PERFORMANCE CRITERIA	**COMPLETED BY STAFF**	
1. Clamps infusion tubing.	Y	N
2. Loosens tape at venipuncture site, while holding needle hub firmly and pull tape toward site.	Y	N
3. Puts non-sterile gloves on.	Y	N
4. Withdraws needle or catheter, placing gauze over IV site.	Y	N
5. Applies firm pressure to site with gauze for 2-3 minutes or until bleeding has stopped.	Y	N
6. If bleeding persists, elevates extremity above body.	Y	N
7. Checks needle or catheter to ensure that it is intact. Reports broken tip or missing pieces to RN.	Y	N
8. Applies sterile dressing (Band-Aid).	Y	N
9. Disposes of equipment in appropriate places according to Safety Standards.	Y	N
10. Records amount of fluid infused.	Y	N
COMMENTS:		

Evaluator_____

NAME _____

UNIT _____

DATE _____

COMPETENCY: Labor and Delivery Scrubbing Techniques		
PERFORMANCE CRITERIA	**COMPLETED BY STAFF**	
1. Performs surgical scrub according to policy.	Y	N
2. Maintains sterile technique throughout procedure.	Y	N
3. Identifies instruments by name which are required for all delivery sets.	Y	N
4. Identifies instruments required for emergency surgical deliveries (Caesarean Sections).	Y	N
5. Distinguishes between suture material needed for closure of routine episiotomies and operative deliveries.	Y	N
6. Counts instruments accurately at the appropriate times.	Y	N
7. Sets up equipment (suction, cautery, etc.) and tests function prior to procedure.	Y	N
8. Sets up table and delivery packs according to unit standard.	Y	N
9. Relieves peers for case completion according to protocol.	Y	N
COMMENTS:		

Evaluator_____

NAME _____

UNIT _____

DATE _____

COMPETENCY: Verification of Last Menstrual Period		
PERFORMANCE CRITERIA	**COMPLETED BY STAFF**	
1. Verifies patient is of child bearing age.	Y	N
2. Establishes LMP.	Y	N
3. If onset of menses greater than 10 days, question patient as to possibility of pregnancy.	Y	N
4. Documents LMP and any other pertinent menstrual information on requestion.	Y	N
5. Responds appropriately to patient questions.	Y	N
COMMENTS:		

Evaluator_____

NAME   _____

UNIT   _____

DATE   _____

COMPETENCY: Screening and Leveling for Risk of Malnutrition		
PERFORMANCE CRITERIA	COMPLETED BY STAFF	
1. The following information is written on the Nutrition Cardex or not available (NA) is written beside it.		
a. name, room number, age, sex	Y	N
b. height, weight	Y	N
c. ideal body weight (IBW)/percent of IBW	Y	N
d. diagnosis	Y	N
e. pertinent medical and surgical history	Y	N
f. lab data	Y	N
1. glucose	Y	N
2. BUN	Y	N
3. creatinine	Y	N
4. sodium	Y	N
5. potassium	Y	N
6. cholesterol	Y	N
7. triglyceride	Y	N
8. albumin	Y	N
9. hemoglobin	Y	N
10. hematocrit	Y	N
11. MCV	Y	N
12. any abnormal lab	Y	N
g. patient's addressograph	Y	N
h. medications - insulin or OHA's only	Y	N
2. Accesses various sources for the above data.	Y	N
3. Accurately levels patient.	Y	N
4. Documents level on Nutrition Cardex.	Y	N
5. Accurately completes screening label.	Y	N
6. Places screening label in appropriate location in the medical record.	Y	N
7. Screening and leveling is completed in a timely manner.	Y	N
COMMENTS:		

Evaluator_____

NAME _____

UNIT _____

DATE _____

COMPETENCY: Maintenance of Hall Power Equipment		
PERFORMANCE CRITERIA	COMPLETED BY STAFF	
1. Cleans hall equipment according to policy.	Y	N
2. Packages equipment properly in preparation for sterilization.	Y	N
COMMENTS:		

Evaluator_____

NAME   _____

UNIT   _____

DATE   _____

COMPETENCY: Immediate Post Operative Pain Management		
PERFORMANCE CRITERIA	**COMPLETED BY STAFF**	

1.   Assesses pain/discomfort level via:
    a. patient complaint of pain
    b. body language interpretation
    c. level of activity - lethargy, sleeping
	Y	N

2. Validates absence of allergy to ordered pain medications.	Y	N
3. Obtains written order for pain medications from anesthesiologist.	Y	N
4. Provides liquids and crackers prior to administration of pain medications.	Y	N
5. Administers correct amount and route of pain medications.	Y	N
6. Documents pain medication administration.	Y	N
7. Observes patient for at least 30 minutes after pain medication administration and documents patient's response to medication.	Y	N
8. If relief is not obtained, requests repeat order from anesthesiologist.	Y	N

9.   Implements additional nursing measures for pain relief:
    a. Change in position
    b. Warm blankets
    c. Limit distractions
    d. Decrease lighting
	Y	N

COMMENTS:		

Evaluator_____

NAME   _____

UNIT   _____

DATE   _____

COMPETENCY: Managing Hypoglycemia in Newborns		
PERFORMANCE CRITERIA	**COMPLETED BY STAFF**	
1. Identifies signs/symptoms of hypoglycemia states in a newborn.	Y	N
2. Identifies newborn at risk for potential hypoglycemia.	Y	N
3. Initiates/identifies appropriate time sequence to be followed for chem protocol for specific newborn scenario.	Y	N
4. Documents/identifies rationale for initiating chem protocol.	Y	N
5. Determines whether results are within normal limits or requires further intervention.	Y	N
6. Identifies high and low critical values.	Y	N
7. Identifies and documents results and plan for corrective action.	Y	N
8. Implements additional chems and interventions according to protocol to maintain euglycemic state (Mother/Baby RN's only).	Y	N
9. Provides parents with teaching regarding purpose of test and subsequent testing.	Y	N
COMMENTS:		

Evaluator_____

NAME   _____

UNIT   _____

DATE   _____

COMPETENCY: Perform Mastectomy Patient Evaluation		
PERFORMANCE CRITERIA	**COMPLETED BY STAFF**	
1. States patient's name on evaluation.	Y	N
2. Identifies date of evaluation.	Y	N
3. Identifies past medical history.	Y	N
4. Identifies current course.	Y	N
5. Performs Musculoskeletal screening.	Y	N
6. Performs daily living skill screening.	Y	N
7. Performs lymphoedema screening.	Y	N
COMMENTS:		

Evaluator_____

NAME   _____

UNIT   _____

DATE   _____

COMPETENCY: Maintenance of Med-Lock (Adult)	
PERFORMANCE CRITERIA	**COMPLETED BY STAFF**
1. Assesses site for pain, weakness, redness, swelling and/or leakage of fluid.	Y N
2. Cleanses diaphragm with alcohol.	Y N
3. Flushes Med-Lock with 1 to 1½ cc of basteriostatic 0.9% normal saline.	Y N
4. Secures Med-Lock to extremity.	Y N
5. Documents flush on Medication Kardex.	Y N
COMMENTS:	

Evaluator_____

NAME _____

UNIT _____

DATE _____

COMPETENCY: Preparation for Menu Distribution		
PERFORMANCE CRITERIA	**COMPLETED**	
	BY STAFF	
1. Writes name on each panel.	Y	N
2. Writes room number on each panel.	Y	N
3. Writes diet on each panel of menu.	Y	N
4. All writing is legible.	Y	N
5. Menu is modified accurately per prescribed diet.	Y	N
6. Appropriate menu is chosen.	Y	N
7. Diet patterns are correct when needed.	Y	N
8. Supplements are written on menu when needed.	Y	N
9. Menu is stapled with modification stamped, when needed.	Y	N
COMMENTS:		

Evaluator_____

NAME   _____

UNIT   _____

DATE   _____

COMPETENCY: Assisting Patient with Menu Selection		
PERFORMANCE CRITERIA	**COMPLETED**	**BY STAFF**
1. Knocks on patient door.	Y	N
2. Greets patient by name: Mr., Mrs., Ms.	Y	N
3. Introduces self.	Y	N
4. Explains his/her purpose in the room.	Y	N
5. Explains the menu.	Y	N
6. Walks patient through the menu.	Y	N
7. Expresses appropriate departure.	Y	N
COMMENTS:		

Evaluator_____

NAME   _____

UNIT   _____

DATE   _____

COMPETENCY: Midas Rex: Set-up and Clean-up		
PERFORMANCE CRITERIA	**COMPLETED BY STAFF**	
1. Assembles all components of Midas Rex System.	Y	N
2. Connects power cord.	Y	N
3. Checks oil level.	Y	N
4. Adjusts lubricant if needed.	Y	N
5. Cleans equipment properly after use.	Y	N
6. Removes felt ring properly.	Y	N
7. Replaces felt ring properly.	Y	N
COMMENTS:		

Evaluator_____

NAME _____

UNIT _____

DATE _____

COMPETENCY: Nasogastric Tube Insertion		
PERFORMANCE CRITERIA	**COMPLETED BY STAFF**	
1. Wash hands.	Y	N
2. Measure length of tube to be inserted and mark tube with a piece of tape.	Y	N
3. Lubricate distal end of tube.	Y	N
4. Don sterile gloves.	Y	N
5. Insert tube into selected nostril.	Y	N
6. Position curved edge of tube downward and direct tube along nostril base.	Y	N
7. When tube reaches posterior nasopharynx, flex patient's neck forward.	Y	N
8. Ask patient to swallow or stimulate swallowing.	Y	N
9. Stop passing the tube at the tape marker.	Y	N
10. Confirm correct position of tube.	Y	N
11. Secure tube in position.	Y	N
12. Secure tube to patient's gown.	Y	N
COMMENTS:		

Evaluator_____

NAME _____

UNIT _____

DATE _____

COMPETENCY: Neonatal Mock Code - Assisting with Endotracheal Intubation		
PERFORMANCE CRITERIA	**COMPLETED BY STAFF**	
1. Selects correct size ET Tube.	Y	N
2. Inserts stylet.	Y	N
3. Selects appropriate size laryngoscope blade.	Y	N
4. Attaches blade to scope and checks light.	Y	N
5. Takes appropriate action if light does not work.	Y	N
6. Cuts strips of tape.	Y	N
7. Obtains bag and mask.	Y	N
8. Prepares tubing with 100% O_2.	Y	N
9. Prepares suction equipment.	Y	N
10. Positions infant.	Y	N
11. Provides free flow O_2.	Y	N
12. Applies laryngeal pressure (if requested).	Y	N
13. Confirms tube placement.	Y	N
14. Secure tube to face (identify steps to secure).	Y	N
COMMENTS:		

Evaluator_____

NAME _____

UNIT _____

DATE _____

COMPETENCY: Neonatal Mock Code - Chest Compressions		
PERFORMANCE CRITERIA	**COMPLETED BY STAFF**	
1. Accurately places fingers on infant's chest.	Y	N
2. Support for infant's back present.	Y	N
3. Compression rate - 120/minute.	Y	N
4. Compression depth - ½" - ¾".	Y	N
5. Keeps fingers on sternum during compression cycle.	Y	N
6. Check heart rate after 30 seconds for 6 seconds.	Y	N
COMMENTS:		

Evaluator_____

NAME   _____

UNIT   _____

DATE   _____

COMPETENCY: Neonatal Mock Code: Use of Resuscitation Bag and Mask	
PERFORMANCE CRITERIA	**COMPLETED BY STAFF**
1. Sets up bag to oxygen source.	Y N
2. Selects mask size	Y N
3. Ensures correct functioning of bag.	Y N
4. Checks infant's position.	Y N
5. Positions bag and mask properly on infant.	Y N
6. Checks seals.	Y N
7. Ventilates 15-30 seconds.	Y N
8. Checks heart rate with stethoscope for 6 seconds.	Y N
COMMENTS:	

Evaluator_____

NAME _____

UNIT _____

DATE _____

COMPETENCY: Neonatal Mock Code: Initial Steps in Resuscitation	
PERFORMANCE CRITERIA	**COMPLETED BY STAFF**
1. Identify under what clinical situations would the need for a resuscitation be anticipated.	Y N
2. Place infant on preheated radiant warmer.	Y N
3. Identify for what reason tracheal suctioning would be done.	Y N
4. Dries infant totally.	Y N
5. Removes wet liner from area.	Y N
6. Slightly extends infant's neck.	Y N
7. Suctions mouth, then nose.	Y N
8. Evaluates respirations.	Y N
9. Evaluates heart rate.	Y N
10. Evaluates color.	Y N
COMMENTS:	

Evaluator_____

NAME   _____

UNIT   _____

DATE   _____

COMPETENCY: Performing a Non-Stress Test		
PERFORMANCE CRITERIA	**COMPLETED BY STAFF**	
1. Explains purpose and procedure to patient/family.	Y	N
2. Validates that gestational ages is appropriate for NST procedure.	Y	N
3. Applies EFM equipment appropriately.	Y	N
4. Positions patient in LLP for optimum tracing.	Y	N
5. Instructs patient how to participate in the NST.	Y	N
6. Maintains patient positioning for continuity of trace patterns.	Y	N
7. Identifies test strip as reactive or non-reactive.	Y	N
8. Implements supportive actions to convert a non-reactive test to a reactive one.	Y	N
9. Distinguishes non-reassuring patterns which need to be reported to the physician.	Y	N
10. Reports to physician appropriately.	Y	N
COMMENTS:		

Evaluator_____

NAME _____

UNIT _____

DATE _____

COMPETENCY: Nursing Care of the Patient With a Non-Viral STD		
PERFORMANCE CRITERIA	**COMPLETED BY STAFF**	
1. Verifies indication for STD treatment.	Y	N
2. Explains name and nature of infection to patient.	Y	N
3. Explains how the disease is transmitted to patient.	Y	N
4. Informs patient of the need for all sexual partners to be treated.	Y	N
5. Provides written directions for partner STD treatment.	Y	N
6. Informs patient of need to abstain from intercourse until test of cure is obtained.	Y	N
7. Medicates patient as ordered.	Y	N
8. Provides written documentation to patient of date of next clinic appointment.	Y	N
9. Provides literature on STD according to Structure Standards.	Y	N
10. Documents provision of care on Sexually Transmitted Disease Protocol (form).	Y	N
COMMENTS:		

Evaluator_____

NAME _____

UNIT _____

DATE _____

COMPETENCY: Sterile technique in the Operating Room		
PERFORMANCE CRITERIA	**COMPLETED BY STAFF**	
1. Scrubs hands and arms for appropriate length of time.	Y	N
2. Places gown and sterile gloves on using sterile technique.	Y	N
3. Creates sterile field by opening sterile packs, linen and instruments correctly.	Y	N
4. Drapes patient correctly for the specific procedure.	Y	N
5. Identifies parameters of sterile field.	Y	N
6. Maintains sterile technique throughout procedure.	Y	N
7. Reports breaks in sterile technique to circulating nurse if it occurs.	Y	N
COMMENTS:		

Evaluator_____

NAME _____
UNIT _____
DATE _____

COMPETENCY: Oral Presentations to Adults		
PERFORMANCE CRITERIA	COMPLETED BY STAFF	
1. Utilizes principles of adult learning.	Y	N
2. Presents information in an organized, systematic manner.	Y	N
3. Uses appropriate verbal communication skills, i.e. projects voice, use of language appropriate for the audience.	Y	N
4. Uses appropriate non-verbal communication i.e. eye contact, body language.	Y	N
5. Encourages questions and discussion when appropriate.	Y	N
6. Uses audiovisual equipment to enhance presentation.	Y	N
7. Uses handouts to help explain presentation.	Y	N
8. Gives examples related to content.	Y	N
COMMENTS:		

Evaluator_____

NAME _____

UNIT _____

DATE _____

COMPETENCY: Ordering Special Food Items		
PERFORMANCE CRITERIA	**COMPLETED**	
	BY STAFF	
1. Places information on correct production sheet.	Y	N
2. Writes patient's name.	Y	N
3. Writes room number.	Y	N
4. Writes in food item requested.	Y	N
5. Writes in correct portion size needed.	Y	N
6. Checks off appropriate column for correct meal.	Y	N
COMMENTS:		

Evaluator_____

NAME _____
UNIT _____
DATE _____

COMPETENCY: Oxygen Tank Changing		
PERFORMANCE CRITERIA	**COMPLETED BY STAFF**	
1. Checks patient's O_2 flow rate.	Y	N
2. Shuts off main valve.	Y	N
3. Removes regulator from empty O_2 tank.	Y	N
4. Places regulator on full O_2 tank and tightens.	Y	N
5. Open main value.	Y	N
6. Sets patient's O_2 flow rate.	Y	N
COMMENTS:		

Evaluator_____

NAME   _____

UNIT   _____

DATE   _____

COMPETENCY: Equipment Set-up for Oxygen Therapy		
PERFORMANCE CRITERIA	**COMPLETED BY STAFF**	
1. Eliminates presence of inflammable chemicals and solution in the environment.	Y	N
2. Assesses patient's respiratory rate and level of consciousness.	Y	N
3. Reminds patient and visitors of NO SMOKING policy and posts "NO SMOKING" signs appropriately.	Y	N
4. Explains procedure to patient	Y	N
5. Fills humidification source initially and periodically throughout therapy.	Y	N
6. Connects tubing to oxygen source and breathing apparatus.	Y	N
COMMENTS:		

Evaluator_____

NAME   _____

UNIT   _____

DATE   _____

COMPETENCY: Oxygen Therapy		
PERFORMANCE CRITERIA	**COMPLETED BY STAFF**	
1. Ascertains appropriate physician order.	Y	N
2. Identifies indications for non-routine precautions.	Y	N
3. Checks device for proper FiO_2/liter flow.	Y	N
4. Checks device at all connections for proper fit/patient comfort.	Y	N
5. Documents procedure appropriately.	Y	N
COMMENTS:		

Evaluator_____

NAME _____

UNIT _____

DATE _____

PATHOLOGY PROCEDURE SELECTED:

COMPETENCY: Performing Selected Pathology Procedures		
PERFORMANCE CRITERIA	**COMPLETED BY STAFF**	
1. Validates receipt of correct specimen type for requested procedure.	Y	N
2. Ensures that specimen is labeled correctly according to department procedure.	Y	N
3. Correctly prepares specimen for specific test procedure as indicated.	Y	N
4. Correctly performs laboratory test according to department procedure.	Y	N
5. Correctly enters result information into the database as indicated.	Y	N
6. Identifies potential inaccuracies in test results if present.	Y	N

7. Validates test procedure and accuracy of results.
   a. Verifies test results after validating correct procedure was followed.
   b. Rechecks procedure again if different results found during validation procedure.
   c. Re-enters accurate results after third testing.
	Y	N

8. Verifies accurate results in database.	Y	N
9. Notifies appropriate care provider of Panic Values, according to department policy.	Y	N
COMMENTS:		
REMEDIAL ACTION:		

Evaluator_____

NAME   _____

UNIT   _____

DATE   _____

COMPETENCY: Solving Procedural Problems in the Pathology Department		
PERFORMANCE CRITERIA	**COMPLETED BY STAFF**	
1. Identifies type of procedural problem:	Y	N
a. mislabeled specimens	Y	N
b. wrong type of specimen for requested procedure	Y	N
c. incorrect sample collection for requested procedure	Y	N
d. incorrect procedural testing	Y	N
e. failed Delta Check	Y	N
f. other	Y	N
2. Collects additional data:	Y	N
a. individual at fault	Y	N
b. actual procedure implemented	Y	N
c. corrective action needed	Y	N
3. Implements corrective action.	Y	N
4. Documents incident if indicated, including:	Y	N
a. names of patient, individual at fault, and person contacted	Y	N
b. date and time of incident	Y	N
c. corrective action taken	Y	N

COMMENTS:

REMEDIAL ACTION:

Evaluator_____

NAME   _____

UNIT   _____

DATE   _____

COMPETENCY: Patient Transport		
PERFORMANCE CRITERIA	**COMPLETED BY STAFF**	
1. Provides clean stretcher and linens for each patient.	Y	N
2. Identifies correct patient for transport.	Y	N
3. Identifies any special instructions from nurse prior to departure from unit.	Y	N
4. Maintains elevated side rails during transport.	Y	N
5. Maintains stabilized IV poles during transport.	Y	N
6. Maintains patients arms and legs in protected positions inside rails.	Y	N
7. Notifies nurse of arrival on unit.	Y	N
COMMENTS:		

Evaluator_____

NAME   _____

UNIT   _____

DATE   _____

COMPETENCY: PCA Pump Set-up		
PERFORMANCE CRITERIA	**COMPLETED BY STAFF**	
1. Checks for physician order.	Y	N
2. Checks with patient for allergies.	Y	N
3. Verifies patient identity.	Y	N
4. Properly sets-up PCA and primary IV.	Y	N
5. Correctly programs PCA infuser.	Y	N
6. Correctly re-programs PCA.	Y	N
7. Correctly trouble-shoots alarms and warning.	Y	N
8. Changes tubing and syringes according to policy.	Y	N
9. Instructs patient on correct use of PCA.	Y	N
10. Documents baseline vital signs, sedation, pain levels, bolus dose and patient education.	Y	N
COMMENTS:		

Evaluator_____

NAME   _____

UNIT   _____

DATE   _____

COMPETENCY: PCA Pump Maintenance	
PERFORMANCE CRITERIA	**COMPLETED BY STAFF**
1. Assesses patient's response to PCA treatment by monitoring respiratory rate, level of consciousness and pain relief at least every 4 hours.	Y N
2. Verifies availability of Narcan within close proximity to patient's bed.	Y N
3. Replaces empty PCA syringe with continuing drug as ordered.	Y N
4. Obtains PCA pump printout every 4 hours.	Y N
5. Changes paper correctly in pump.	Y N
6. Maintains pump's electrical supply and grounding source according to safety standards.	Y N
COMMENTS:	

Evaluator_____

NAME _____
UNIT _____
DATE _____

COMPETENCY: Pediatric Speech and Language Screening		
PERFORMANCE CRITERIA	**COMPLETED**	
	BY STAFF	
1. Introduces self to child and family.	Y	N
2. Describes procedure to child and family.	Y	N
3. Chooses age appropriate screening tool.	Y	N
4. Completely fills out screening tool.	Y	N
5. Makes recommendations for therapy if indicated.	Y	N
6. Schedules evaluation appointment.	Y	N
7. Documents screening in medical record.	Y	N
COMMENTS:		

Evaluator_____

NAME _____

UNIT _____

DATE _____

COMPETENCY: Preparing Patients for Pelvic Exams		
PERFORMANCE CRITERIA	**COMPLETED BY STAFF**	
1. Assists patient onto examination table.	Y	N
2. Appropriately drapes patient for specific procedure.	Y	N
3. Assists patient in proper position and use of stirrups.	Y	N
4. Properly disposes of linens and table covers following examination.	Y	N
COMMENTS:		

Evaluator_____

NAME _____

UNIT _____

DATE _____

COMPETENCY: Management of Perinatal Loss Support Program		
PERFORMANCE CRITERIA	**COMPLETED BY STAFF**	
1. Assesses needed for referral to "Mercy Cares" program.	Y	N
2. Initiates "Mercy Cares" procedures/paper work as soon as patient arrives on unit.	Y	N
3. Serves as patient advocate by providing privacy and support.	Y	N
4. Answers questions regarding loss from patient and family.	Y	N
5. Provides patient and family with appropriate literature.	Y	N
6. Provides environment for patient/family to state feelings concerning loss.	Y	N
7. Refers patient/family to appropriate care staff available for support.	Y	N
8. Places "Mercy Cares" card on patient's door.	Y	N

9. Notifies the following departments/people within 2 hrs of loss:
   a. "Mercy Cares" Coordinator
   b. Pastoral Care
   c. Social Work
	Y	N

10. Verifies information completed by physician immediately after loss.	Y	N
11. Explains burial options to patient and family.	Y	N
12. Enables patient/family to spend time with fetus/neonate after loss.	Y	N
13. Offers infant's memorabilia packet to patient at discharge. If patient chooses not to accept packet, sends it to "Mercy Cares" Coordinator.	Y	N
14. Takes fetus/neonate to morgue/pathology.	Y	N
COMMENTS:		

Evaluator_____

NAME   _____

UNIT   _____

DATE   _____

COMPETENCY: Supporting a Family After Perinatal Loss.	
PERFORMANCE CRITERIA	**COMPLETED BY STAFF**
1. Provides privacy for patient and family.	Y N
2. Recognizes significance of "Mercy Cares" card on patient's door.	Y N
3. Provides patient/family adequate time with fetus/neonate after loss.	Y N
4. Acts as patient advocate.	Y N
5. Provides environment for patient to state feelings concerning loss.	Y N
6. Provides environment for family to discuss loss as appropriate.	Y N
7. Notifies R.N. of patient needs when verbalized.	Y N
8. Provides comfort measures p.r.n.	Y N
COMMENTS:	

Evaluator_____

NAME _____

UNIT _____

DATE _____

COMPETENCY: Verification of Pregnancy		
PERFORMANCE CRITERIA	**COMPLETED BY STAFF**	
1. Establishes date of LMP.	Y	N

2. Determines appropriate method for verifying pregnancy status:
  a. If menses are more than 10 days late or patient gives history of irregular bleeding, orders serum HCG.
  b. If LMP indicates gestation of 12 weeks or more, attempts to listen for FHT via Doppler.
  c. If unable to locate FHT for patient with indicated gestation of 12 weeks or more, orders serum HCG.
	Y	N

3. Provides written instructions on how patient can obtain serum HCG results.	Y	N
4. If pregnancy is verified by positive serum HCG or presence of FHT, arranges for prenatal care.	Y	N
5. Documents process of pregnancy verification utilizing Pregnancy Screening Form correctly.	Y	N
COMMENTS:		

Evaluator_____

NAME   _____

UNIT   _____

DATE   _____

COMPETENCY: **Manages Quality Control Program for Nuclear Medicine Department**		
PERFORMANCE CRITERIA	**COMPLETED BY STAFF**	
1. Reviews daily QC documentation	Y	N
a. camera floods	Y	N
b. constancy sheets	Y	N
c. film processor function	Y	N
d. freezer, refrigerator, water bath temperature	Y	N
2. Implements action plans for unusual QC findings.	Y	N
3. Reports unusual findings to department director.	Y	N
4. Documents action taken for unusual QC findings on individual QC worksheets.	Y	N
COMMENTS:		

Evaluator_____

NAME   _____

UNIT   _____

DATE   _____

COMPETENCY: Prepares, Calibrates and Administers Radiopharmaceutical in a Aseptic Manner	
PERFORMANCE CRITERIA	**COMPLETED BY STAFF**
1. Washes hands and puts on non-sterile gloves.	Y N
2. Selects the proper kit with the reagent to be prepared.	Y N
3. Checks the expiration date on the reagent vial.	Y N
4. Using a sterile technique, shields syringe.	Y N
5. Aseptically add 2-8 ml. of Tc99m to the vial.	Y N
6. Place fitted cover onto the lead shield, swirl the contents for 1 minutes and let stand.	Y N
7. Record the time and date of preparation, the volume, activity and calibration of the Tc99m injection added.	Y N
8. Store the finished product in a lead shield at room temperature.	Y N
COMMENTS:	

Evaluator_____

NAME _____

UNIT _____

DATE _____

COMPETENCY: Respiratory Therapy Unit Rounds - Critical Care Unit		
PERFORMANCE CRITERIA	**COMPLETED BY STAFF**	
1. Checks charts for Respiratory Orders.	Y	N
2. Checks results of latest ABG's and CXR's.	Y	N
3. Checks breath sounds for proper tube placement (ventilator patients).	Y	N
4. Checks ventilator circuit.	Y	N
5. Checks wiring on equipment for potential hazards.	Y	N
6. Charts all ventilator parameters.	Y	N
7. Changes Closed-System Suction Catheter every day.	Y	N
8. Obtains weaning parameters on all appropriate patients.	Y	N
9. Measures Cuff Pressure.	Y	N
10. Checks all Oxygen Therapy.	Y	N
11. Checks Pulse Oximetry Data, including site and alarm limits.	Y	N
12. Completes all appropriate documentation.	Y	N
COMMENTS:		

Evaluator_____

NAME   _____

UNIT   _____

DATE   _____

COMPETENCY: Respiratory Therapy Unit Rounds - Neonatal Intensive Care Unit		
PERFORMANCE CRITERIA	**COMPLETED BY STAFF**	
1. Checks charts for Respiratory Orders.	Y	N
2. Checks ventilator circuit.	Y	N
3. Checks wiring on equipment for potential hazards.	Y	N
4. Charts all ventilator parameters.	Y	N
5. Checks all Oxygen Therapy devices.	Y	N
6. Checks Pulse Oximetry Data, including site and alarm limits.	Y	N
7. Completes all appropriate documentation.	Y	N
COMMENTS:		

Evaluator_____

NAME _____

UNIT _____

DATE _____

COMPETENCY: Deliver Sequential Pump Therapy		
PERFORMANCE CRITERIA	COMPLETED BY STAFF	
1. Performs girth measurements.	Y	N
2. Performs volumetric measurement.	Y	N
3. Performs blood pressure assessment.	Y	N
4. Positions upper extremity.	Y	N
5. Dons sleeve correctly.	Y	N
6. Sets appropriate pressure.	Y	N
7. Performs post treatment edema measurements.	Y	N
COMMENTS:		

Evaluator_____

233

NAME _____
UNIT _____
DATE _____

COMPETENCY: Utilization of Stackhouse Smoke Evacuator		
PERFORMANCE CRITERIA	**COMPLETED BY STAFF**	
1. Obtains new filter canister and tubing for each case.	Y	N
2. Connects tubing to canister on front.	Y	N
3. Holds tubing close to operative area and collects all smoke.	Y	N
4. At conclusion of case, connects both ends of tubing into a closed loop.	Y	N
5. Caps both ends of canister.	Y	N
6. Discards closed tubing system and closed canister into red bags and places bags in appropriate disposal facilities according to policy.	Y	N
COMMENTS:		

Evaluator_____

NAME   _____

UNIT   _____

DATE   _____

COMPETENCY: Performing an Intrinsic Tc99m Flood on the Sophy X-Camera		
PERFORMANCE CRITERIA	**COMPLETED BY STAFF**	
1. Washes hands and puts on non-sterile gloves.	Y	N
2. Draws 200 uCi of Tc99m radioactive material up in a syringe.	Y	N
3. Checks the dose in the radioisotope dose calibrator.	Y	N
4. Places the dose in a lead pig and continue to the Sophy Camera X.	Y	N
5. Removes collimator and position camera properly.	Y	N
6. Peaks the camera in on Tc99m 140/20.	Y	N
7. Performs two floods (1-1 millions counts; 1-4 million counts).	Y	N
8. Accurately reads test results - checking for uniformity & sensitivity.	Y	N
9. Replaces collimator on camera - up & ready.	Y	N
10. Documents results & notifies senior technologist of abnormal results.	Y	N
COMMENTS:		

Evaluator_____

NAME _____

UNIT _____

DATE _____

COMPETENCY: Sterilizing Equipment	
PERFORMANCE CRITERIA	COMPLETED BY STAFF
1. Identifies the type of sterilization needed for specific equipment (e.g. gas vs. steam).	Y N
2. Sends equipment which needs gas sterilization to Central Supply.	Y N
3. Steam sterilizes equipment using adequate pressure and temperature.	Y N
4. Challenges sterilizers using correct sequence.	Y N
5. Labels sterilized kits appropriately.	Y N
COMMENTS:	

Evaluator_____

NAME _____

UNIT _____

DATE _____

COMPETENCY: Maintenance of Suction during an Operative Procedure		
PERFORMANCE CRITERIA	**COMPLETED BY STAFF**	
1. Assembles appropriate equipment.	Y	N
2. Accurately connects all tubing before procedure.	Y	N
3. Disconnects tubing, maintaining universal precautions, after procedure.	Y	N
4. Caps all containers after procedure.	Y	N
5. Disposes of canister contents according to unit standards.	Y	N
6. Prepares another system for next procedure.	Y	N
COMMENTS:		

Evaluator_____

NAME _____

UNIT _____

DATE _____

COMPETENCY: Endotracheal Tube Suctioning (NICU)		
PERFORMANCE CRITERIA	COMPLETED BY STAFF	
1. Sets-up equipment and supplies correctly.	Y	N
2. Selects appropriate sized suction catheter.	Y	N
3. Ensures that ET tube is anchored securely.	Y	N
4. Auscultates lungs prior to procedure.	Y	N
5. Identifies appropriate length of catheter to be inserted.	Y	N
6. Suctions infant according to unit policy, not to exceed 10 seconds per suction pass.	Y	N
7. Ambu-bags infant at correct manometer pressure after each suction pass until color, HR and SaO_2 return to baseline.	Y	N
8. Repeats procedure up to 2 times more p.r.n.	Y	N
9. Assesses need for mouth suctioning.	Y	N
10. Auscultates lungs after procedure.	Y	N
11. Reports any bradycardia during suctioning to Neonatal Nurse Practitioner.	Y	N
12. Documents procedure according to unit policy.	Y	N
COMMENTS:		

Evaluator_____

NAME   _____

UNIT   _____

DATE   _____

COMPETENCY: Oropharyngeal Suctioning		
PERFORMANCE CRITERIA	**COMPLETED BY STAFF**	
1. Maintains clean technique throughout the procedure.	Y	N
2. Explains procedure to patient.	Y	N
3. Position patient appropriately = conscious patient: Semi-Fowler's with head to one side; unconscious patient: lateral position.	Y	N
4. Properly drapes patient.	Y	N
5. Sets suction pressure appropriately.	Y	N
6. Dons sterile gloves and attaches catheter to suction unit. Tests suction catheter patency.	Y	N
7. Accurately identifies length of catheter tube to be inserted.	Y	N
8. Lubricates catheter tip with water or sterile lubricating gel. Insert lubricated tip into side of mouth with suction.	Y	N
9. Suctions mouth correctly for no more than 15 seconds.	Y	N
10. Flushes catheter after each suction attempt. Continues additional 15 second attempts until passage is clear.	Y	N
11. Encourages patient to breath deeply and cough between suction attempts.	Y	N
12. Provides oral hygiene after procedure.	Y	N
13. Disposes of equipment correctly according to Universal Precautions.	Y	N
14. Reports amount, color, consistency and odor of sputum to nurse.	Y	N
COMMENTS:		

Evaluator_____

NAME _____

UNIT _____

DATE _____

COMPETENCY: Performs Stress Test		
PERFORMANCE CRITERIA	COMPLETED BY STAFF	
1. Instructs patient about test to be performed including complications/side effects.	Y	N
2. Obtains consent forms.	Y	N
3. Takes and records patient Blood Pressure.	Y	N
4. Performs EKG.	Y	N
5. Preps patient according to procedure.	Y	N
6. Places electrodes correctly.	Y	N
7. Hooks patient to treadmill.	Y	N
8. Check Blood Pressure.	Y	N
9. Instruct patient if appropriate in proper treadmill operation to insure patient's safety.	Y	N
10. Watch patient and monitor during test.	Y	N
11. Monitor and record Blood Pressure during test.	Y	N
12. Help patient off treadmill when test is finished.	Y	N
13. Accompany patient to Nuclear Medicine.	Y	N
14. Send report to patient's physician.	Y	N
COMMENTS:		

Evaluator_____

NAME _____

UNIT _____

DATE _____

COMPETENCY: Maintenance of Thermodilution Catheters (Swan Ganz)		
PERFORMANCE CRITERIA	**COMPLETED BY STAFF**	
1. Observes for changes in PAP or PCWP waveform. If changes occur the nurse should:	Y	N
a. Check patient status.	Y	N
b. Recalibrate and check scale.	Y	N
c. Deflate catheter balloon.	Y	N
d. Check all connections and pressure bag.	Y	N
e. Flush the catheter.	Y	N
f. Observe pressurized system for air bubbles.	Y	N
g. Change the patient's position.	Y	N
h. Tell the patient to cough, if possible.	Y	N
2. Notify the physician if these measures are unsuccessful in correcting the problem.	Y	N
3. Nurses are responsible for obtaining patient parameters during the first 8 hours after insertion as follows: a. Q 1 HR: PAP, mean PCWP, CVP, SVO2 with Opticath; then Q 2 HRS. b. Q 2 HRS: CO, SVR; then Q 4 HRS.	Y	N
COMMENTS:		

Evaluator_____

NAME _____

UNIT _____

DATE _____

COMPETENCY: Teaching Injection Technique		
PERFORMANCE CRITERIA	**COMPLETED BY STAFF**	
1. Assesses patient/family knowledge base.	Y	N
2. Verifies physician order.	Y	N
3. Teaches injection technique according to unit policy.	Y	N
4. Explains the pharmacology of the medication.	Y	N
5. Observes the technique by return demonstration until patient/family verbalizes comfort in performing the skill independently.	Y	N
COMMENTS:		

Evaluator_____

NAME _____

UNIT _____

DATE _____

COMPETENCY: Telemetry Lead Placement		
PERFORMANCE CRITERIA	**COMPLETED**	
	BY STAFF	
1. Explains procedure to patient.	Y	N
2. Prepares skin with Skin Prep and allows prep to dry if needed.	Y	N
3. Applies electrodes according to policy.	Y	N
4. Attaches leads via Lead II configuration.	Y	N
COMMENTS:		

Evaluator_____

NAME _____

UNIT _____

DATE _____

COMPETENCY: Tympanic Temperatures		
PERFORMANCE CRITERIA	**COMPLETED BY STAFF**	
1. Participant selects Tympanic mode.	Y	N
2. Participant removes machine form charger and waits for "ready" reading.	Y	N
3. Participant places disposable probe cover on probe.	Y	N
4. Participant places probe at ear canal and seals outer opening.	Y	N
5. Participant presses scan button on probe handle.	Y	N
6. Participant waits for beep to sound and red light to illuminate temperature.	Y	N
7. Participant identifies temperature.	Y	N
COMMENTS:		

Evaluator_____

NAME _____

UNIT _____

DATE _____

COMPETENCY: Testing Urine by Dipstick		
PERFORMANCE CRITERIA	**COMPLETED BY STAFF**	
1. Wash hands and put on non-sterile gloves.	Y	N
2. Choose correct dipstick for type of test.	Y	N
3. Check expiration date on dipstick bottle.	Y	N
4. Dip dipstick in urine until entire test pad is wet.	Y	N
5. Tap dipstick on side of specimen container.	Y	N
6. Compare test strip to Key within 3 seconds of required time for testing.	Y	N
7. Accurately reads test results.	Y	N
8. Documents results and notifies R.N. of abnormal results.	Y	N
COMMENTS:		

Evaluator_____

NAME _____

UNIT _____

DATE _____

COMPETENCY: Maintenance of Tourniquet Tank		
PERFORMANCE CRITERIA	**COMPLETED BY STAFF**	
1. Assembles all equipment.	Y	N
2. Opens tank appropriately.	Y	N
3. Tests tourniquet prior to use, according to unit standards.	Y	N
4. Turns tank off after use.	Y	N
5. Disassembles and changes tank when empty.	Y	N
COMMENTS:		

Evaluator_____

NAME _____

UNIT _____

DATE _____

COMPETENCY: Tracheostomy Care		
PERFORMANCE CRITERIA	**COMPLETED BY STAFF**	
1. Assesses stoma for redness, swelling or drainage.	Y	N
2. Assembles appropriate equipment, including hydrogen peroxide and sterile water, to bedside table.	Y	N
3. Washes hands and pujts on sterile gloves.	Y	N
4. Suctions trachea and pharynx thoroughly using aseptic technique.	Y	N
5. Removes inner cannula of tracheostomy, cleans with hydrogen peroxide and rinses with sterile water. Dries cannula with sterile gauze. Replaces inner cannula.	Y	N
6. Cleans stoma area with peroxide, removing crusted secretions.	Y	N
7. Dries stoma area with gauze sponges.	Y	N
8. Applies antiseptic ointments to stoma as ordered.	Y	N
9. Changes tracheostomy ties maintaining secure stabilization of tracheostomy throughout the procedure.	Y	N
10. Documents performance of procedure, stoma assessment, nature of secretions and patient's tolerance of procedure.	Y	N
COMMENTS:		

Evaluator_____

NAME _____

UNIT _____

DATE _____

COMPETENCY: Traction Set-Up		
PERFORMANCE CRITERIA	**COMPLETED BY STAFF**	
1. Chooses correct traction apparatus according to physician order.	Y	N
2. Places traction frame correctly and tightly onto bed frame.	Y	N
3. Applies ordered amount of weight onto traction apparatus.	Y	N
4. Ensures that weights are free-hanging away from bed.	Y	N
5. Places call button and trapeze within reach of patient.	Y	N
COMMENTS:		

Evaluator_____

NAME   _____

UNIT   _____

DATE   _____

COMPETENCY: Demonstrate Competency in Ultrasound Unit Use		
PERFORMANCE CRITERIA	**COMPLETED BY STAFF**	
1. Therapist prepares patient with appropriate positioning/draping.	Y	N
2. Therapist prepares skin area with appropriate conductive agent.	Y	N
3. Therapist chooses appropriate ultrasound head.	Y	N
4. Therapist sets times.	Y	N
5. Therapist sets frequency.	Y	N
6. Therapist initiates treatment while adjusting intensity.	Y	N
COMMENTS:		

Evaluator_____

NAME _____

UNIT _____

DATE _____

COMPETENCY: Ability to Deliver Ultrasound Therapy		
PERFORMANCE CRITERIA	**COMPLETED BY STAFF**	
1. Performs musculoskeletal assessment.	Y	N
2. Determines the need for Ultrasound Therapy.	Y	N
3. Determines the parameters for Ultrasound machine.	Y	N
4. Sets parameters on Ultrasound machine.	Y	N
5. Applies Ultrasound gel.	Y	N
6. Initiates Ultrasound treatment.	Y	N
7. Continues motion of Ultrasound head during Ultrasound treatment.	Y	N
8. After Ultrasound treatment, cleans treatment area with alcohol.	Y	N
9. Cleans Ultrasound head with alcohol.	Y	N
10. Reassesses patient for efforts of treatment.	Y	N
COMMENTS:		

Evaluator_____

NAME   _____

UNIT   _____

DATE   _____

COMPETENCY: Ultrasound - Amniocentsis & Thoracentesis Procedures		
PERFORMANCE CRITERIA	COMPLETED BY STAFF	
1. Calls patient by name.	Y	N
2. Verifies clinical information.	Y	N
3. Changes patient.	Y	N
4. Educates patient regarding procedure.	Y	N
5. Documents education.	Y	N
6. Obtains signed consent to treatment.	Y	N
7. Properly sets up appropriate tray and/or equipment using sterile technique.	Y	N
8. Locates and accurately marks fluid pocket.	Y	N
9. Hard copies on film.	Y	N
10. Rescans patient post-procedure.	Y	N
11. Documents all pertinent information.	Y	N
COMMENTS:		

Evaluator_____

NAME _____

UNIT _____

DATE _____

COMPETENCY: Ultrasound - Carotid Dopplers		
PERFORMANCE CRITERIA	**COMPLETED BY STAFF**	
1. Calls patient by name.	Y	N
2. Verifies clinical indications and exam ordered.	Y	N
3. Educates patient regarding exam.	Y	N
4. Performs procedure according to department procedures and protocols.	Y	N
5. Records procedure on hard copy according to department protocols.	Y	N
6. Documents all pertinent information on Carotid Worksheet.	Y	N
7. Documents all pertinent information in Meditech System.	Y	N
COMMENTS:		

Evaluator_____

NAME _____

UNIT _____

DATE _____

COMPETENCY: Ultrasound - Verification of Patient History		
PERFORMANCE CRITERIA	**COMPLETED BY STAFF**	
1. Validate exam ordered and clinical indications.	Y	N
2. Reviews results of prior exams that are pertinent to current exam.	Y	N
3. Reads patient history.	Y	N
4. Reviews prior ultrasound scan to ensure same technique is used.	Y	N
5. Documents all pertinent information.	Y	N
COMMENTS:		

Evaluator_____

NAME _____
UNIT _____
DATE _____

COMPETENCY: Venipuncture		
PERFORMANCE CRITERIA	**COMPLETED BY STAFF**	
1. Correctly identifies patient.	Y	N
2. Verifies ordered test.	Y	N
3. Selects and assembles appropriate equipment.	Y	N
4. Washes hands thoroughly.	Y	N
5. Explains procedure to client when appropriate.	Y	N
6. Selects the proper vein for collection.	Y	N
7. Utilizes sterile technique in performing collection.	Y	N
8. Performs venipuncture utilizing appropriate technique with:		
a. Vacutainer	Y	N
b. Butterfly	Y	N
c. Syringe (when appropriate)	Y	N
9. Labels all specimens correctly.	Y	N
10. Demonstrates appropriate technique when drawing for special procedure.		
a. Multipe samples	Y	N
b. Blood Bank specimen's	Y	N
c. Blood cultures	Y	N
11. Disposes of venipunture equipment in appropriate containers.	Y	N

12. Provides appropriate post-Phlebotomy care of patient
    a. Removes tourniquet
    b. Removes needle
    c. Bandages site
	Y	N

COMMENTS:		

Evaluator_____

254

NAME _____

UNIT _____

DATE _____

COMPETENCY: Venipuncture for IV Contrast Administration		
PERFORMANCE CRITERIA	**COMPLETED BY STAFF**	
1. Explains procedure to patient.	Y	N
2. Selects proper vein.	Y	N
3. Performs venipuncture utilizing proper technique.	Y	N
4. Successfully performs venipuncture with no more than 2 attempts in 75% of cases.	Y	N
5. Disposes of needle and syringe in appropriate containers.	Y	N
COMMENTS:		

Evaluator_____

NAME _____

UNIT _____

DATE _____

COMPETENCY: Use of Video Camera		
PERFORMANCE CRITERIA	**COMPLETED BY STAFF**	
1. Gathers needed equipment.	Y	N
2. Positions equipment to facilitate optimum video taping.	Y	N
3. Connects equipment appropriately.	Y	N
4. Runs audio and visual tests to insure proper operation of equipment.	Y	N
5. Instructs presenter on video taping procedure.	Y	N
6. Completes video taping.	Y	N
7. Disassembles equipment and returns to proper storage area.	Y	N
COMMENTS:		

Evaluator_____

NAME   _____

UNIT   _____

DATE   _____

COMPETENCY: Management of the Violent Patient		
PERFORMANCE CRITERIA	COMPLETED BY STAFF	
1. Secures adequate assistance from other staff.	Y	N
2. Removes any personal articles which may be used as weapons by patient (e.g. pens, stethoscopes, etc.).	Y	N
3. Decides on exact role of each staff member prior to approaching patient (e.g. who will take to lead and talk to patient, who will be responsible for each limb).	Y	N
4. Agrees upon signal for approaching patient.	Y	N
5. Approaches patient with restraints in hand.	Y	N
6. Upon signal from Team Leader, proceeds to take patient safely to the floor.	Y	N
7. Carries patient to bed.	Y	N
8. Applies restraints.	Y	N
COMMENTS:		

Evaluator_____

257

NAME _____

UNIT _____

DATE _____

COMPETENCY: Vision Screening Using Titmus Tester	
PERFORMANCE CRITERIA	**COMPLETED BY STAFF**
1. Control environment and eliminates distractions.	Y N
2. Chooses age-appropriate chart.	Y N
3. Adjusts instrument body to comfort level of patient.	Y N
4. Places patient's forehead on headrest.	Y N
5. Performs screening using procedure guidelines outline in Structure Standard.	Y N
6. Explains to patient that the E's are in different directions with each turn.	Y N
7. Records findings.	Y N
COMMENTS:	

Evaluator_____

NAME _____

UNIT _____

DATE _____

COMPETENCY: Taking Vital Signs		
PERFORMANCE CRITERIA	**COMPLETED BY STAFF**	
RESPIRATIONS		
1. Participant watches chest rise and fall or listens via stethoscope for at least 30 seconds (60 seconds for a newborn).	Y	N
2. Participant accurately determines the respiratory rate (accurately means within 2 breaths/minute of the rate measured by the evaluator).	Y	N
TEMPERATURE		
1. Participant asks client if they have had anything to eat or drink within the last 15 minutes.	Y	N
2. Participant utilizes the correct probe (blue tip for oral, red for rectal).	Y	N
3. Participant utilizes probe coves correctly (proper fit, Universal Precautions).	Y	N
4. Participant waits for the IVAC to beep to identify the temp.	Y	N
RADIAL PULSE		
1. Participant locates the radial pulse on the inner aspect of the wrist above the thumb.	Y	N
2. Participant palpates the radial pulse using two or three fingers but not their thumb.	Y	N
3. Participant counts pulse for at least 30 seconds.	Y	N
4. Participant accurately determines the pulse (accurately means within 4 beats/minute of the rate measured by the evaluator).	Y	N
APICAL PULSE		
1. Participant places stethoscope over the apex of the heart.	Y	N
2. Participant counts pulse for 60 seconds.	Y	N
3. Participant accurately determines the pulse (accurately means within 4 beats/minute of the rate measured by the evaluator).	Y	N
BLOOD PRESSURE		
1. Participant identifies baseline Blood Pressure.	Y	N
2. Participant places cuff correctly over artery.	Y	N
3. Participant places stethoscope correctly over brachial pulse.	Y	N
4. Participant pumps BP cuff to 170 mm HG or 40 mm Hg above baseline.	Y	N
5. Participant accurately identifies systolic BP (accurately means within 4 mm Hg of the level measured by the evaluator).	Y	N
6. Participant accurately identifies diastolic BP (accurately means within 4 mm Hg of the level measured by the evaluator).	Y	N
DOCUMENTATION		
1. Appropriately documents all VS according to Unit Structure Standards (attach graph).	Y	N
COMMENTS:		

Evaluator_____

NAME _____

UNIT _____

DATE _____

COMPETENCY: Vital Sign Measurement via Electronic Instrument		
PERFORMANCE CRITERIA	**COMPLETED BY STAFF**	
1. Participant identifies baseline blood pressure.	Y	N
2. Participant sets selection switch based on baseline blood pressure.	Y	N
3. Participant places cuff correctly over artery.	Y	N
4. Participant presses the on/off switch and instructs the patient to relax, remain still, and not to talk during the measurement.	Y	N
5. Participant initiates a measurement cycle by pressing the start/reset switch.	Y	N
6. Participant reads the BP and Pulse from the display.	Y	N
7. Participant removes cuff and presses the on/off switch to turn the machine off.	Y	N
8. Participant accurately documents the BP and Pulse according to unit standards.	Y	N
COMMENTS:		

Evaluator_____

NAME   _____

UNIT   _____

DATE   _____

COMPETENCY: Waste Removal		
PERFORMANCE CRITERIA	**COMPLETED BY STAFF**	
1. Disposes of solid wastes in red bags using universal precautions.	Y	N
2. Disposes of liquid wastes in specified containers using universal precautions.	Y	N
3. Disposes of soiled linens appropriately using universal precautions.	Y	N
COMMENTS:		

Evaluator_____

NAME   _____

UNIT   _____

DATE   _____

COMPETENCY: Outpatient Documentation for Physicial Therapy		
PERFORMANCE CRITERIA	**COMPLETED BY STAFF**	
1. Therapist writes a progress note for each treatment listed on the computer read out.	Y	N
2. Rx kept timely - every 30 days.	Y	N
3. PTA assures re-assessment by PT every 10 visits/30 days.	Y	N
4. PTA's treatment is reproducible based on daily progress note.	Y	N
5. PTA includes treatment parameters (for all equipment used during treatment).	Y	N
6. PTA's notes are fully legible.	Y	N
7. PTA gives PT instruction in home program (activities and reps).	Y	N
8. PTA signs each note.	Y	N
9. PTA assures presence of patient progress notes and discharge summary to MD by their presence in chart.	Y	N
COMMENTS:		

Evaluator_____

CHAPTER 5

UNIVERSAL FORMS

Chapter 5

UNIVERSAL FORMS

This chapter includes generic versions of the forms utilized in the competency assessment program described in this book. These forms are designed to guide the user through the development of a competency assessment program, from development of a departmental plan through monitoring of compliance rates and evaluation of clinical performance during orientation of new staff. The forms include:

* A *Department Plan* document structured to aid in the identification of required competency assessments for each level of staff.

* A *Competency Worksheet* providing a structure for detailing the steps in any given competency.

* A *Compliance Summary* form for establishing a mechanism to monitor staff compliance rates with the Assessment Program.

* A *Clinical Performance Evaluation Tool* for guiding and evaluating the staff member's performance during orientation.

Competency Attainment Record

Name of Staff Member	Competency & Date									

CLINICAL PERFORMANCE EVALUATION

NAME	HAVE HAD EXPERIENCE. FEEL COMFORTABLE DOING	LIMITED EXPERIENCE. ASSISTANCE NEEDED	DEMONSTRATED WITH ASSISTANCE	MANAGED INDEPENDENTLY	
	To be Completed be Orientee		To be Completed be Preceptor		

266

NAME	To be Completed be Orientee		To be Completed be Preceptor		
	HAVE HAD EXPERIENCE FEEL COMFORTABLE DOING	LIMITED EXPERIENCE ASSISTANCE NEEDED	DEMONSTRATED WITH ASSISTANCE	MANAGED INDEPENDENTLY	

Recommendations:

Items that will need further assistant with are:

ORIENTEE: _____

PRECEPTOR: _____

MANAGER/DESIGNATE: _____

Competency Assessment Plan for:_____

Policy/Procedure/Protocol

Distribution: Unit Specific

Purpose: To assure that all staff members in the _____ meet the identified competencies established for their job description.

Policy: The following competencies/educational activities will be assessed annually for each staff member:

1. **Position Title**

    Competency Assessments:
    1.
    2.
    3.

    Educational Activities:
    1.
    2.
    3.

2. **Position Title**

    Competency Assessments:
    1.
    2.
    3.

    Educational Activities:
    1.
    2.
    3.

3. **Position Title**

    Competency Assessments:
    1.
    2.
    3.

    Educational Activities:
    1.
    2.
    3.

NAME _____
UNIT _____
DATE _____

COMPETENCY:		
PERFORMANCE CRITERIA	**COMPLETED**	
	BY STAFF	
	Y	N
	Y	N
	Y	N
	Y	N
	Y	N
	Y	N
	Y	N
	Y	N
	Y	N
	Y	N
	Y	N
	Y	N
	Y	N
	Y	N

COMMENTS:

Evaluator_____

INDEX